MAXIMIZING FERTILITY

Proven guide to a successful pregnancy,
reproductive health and preventing miscarriages.
Maximize your fertility through charting while
maintaining
a healthy diet and lifestyle.

Dana Nelson

Table of Contents

Introduction

Hello,

I want to take a moment to thank you for downloading this guide to your own fertility awareness. I know that, by purchasing this book, you might have a lot on your mind about your own chances of conceiving. You are not alone. There are millions of other women like you that are blind about their own fertility.

It seems odd, does it not? We live in an era of information, yet topics regarding women's health are so often shielded from the general public. This leaves women at a disadvantage when it comes to understanding their own bodies — especially when it comes to conceiving babies.

In purchasing this guide, you are probably curious about your own fertility. Perhaps you have had a devastating loss or you are struggling to conceive, and you have turned to this guide to advice. It does not matter where you sit in life on your journey to fertility awareness, this guide will carry you through the rough waters into an arena of enlightenment.

What is fertility awareness exactly? While this question may seem simple enough to answer at first glance, there are a lot of different answers you might come up with yourself. Fertility awareness involves two parts. The first is being aware of your body's cycles and when you are ovulating in an effort to avoid pregnancy. The second is to be aware of when your body is in its prime moments for a successful conception. Sounds easy enough, right? Being aware of your body and its constant changes can be challenging for any woman, especially when you are new to the game.

My goal for you by the end of this guide is to arm you with the tools that you need in order to better understand your cycle and the needs of your body. My objective is to never undermine the struggles you might have gone through before picking up this guide but to help you in seeking further knowledge about yourself.

So, you want to learn about fertility! This guide is the solution to all of the problems that you might be bearing on your own (such as miscarriage and conceiving struggles). You will be able to chart your own cycles by the time you have read the last word in this guide. For those of you who are reading this guide and suffer from deeper tragedies such as miscarriages, my goal is that you will be able to achieve fertility through understanding, charting, and following your cycle. Your diet also plays a huge component in your fertility, and I will expand on that later in this guide so that you are armed with all the knowledge you need to successfully conceive!

Miscarriages are a tremendously difficult time in any woman's life. There are no words for the loss of a baby that you desired. Hopefully, you will find words of comfort through this guide if you have suffered such a loss. I also hope that you find methods that will help you avoid potential future miscarriages as well. Your fertility is your own personal journey of self-discovery and understanding, and this will make all the difference on your path to becoming a mother!

I have been in your shoes before — unaware of my own body's hormonal changes and what they meant. I suffered a devastating loss. After being told that there was nothing I could have done to prevent the loss of my baby, I knew that there was more to it, I simply was not educated about it yet. I sought to change that fact, so I went to school. I devoured all of the information that I could about women and our bodies. I was shocked at how much information the female population misses out on simply because we are not being taught. I knew this had to change. I knew there were other women who needed guidance as I did.

In this guide, chapters one to three will explore your fertility and your cycle. I want you to get comfortable with the different stages that your body goes through and to begin thinking about how you can chart and keep track of your body's changes. It takes time to adjust to viewing your body in a different way, but we are going to take it slow and in-depth so that you have time to adjust. The information in these chapters will range from understanding more about fertility awareness and how it affects you, to understanding what the different phases of your cycle are and how to keep track of them to maximize your fertility window!

As you dig into chapters four and five, I tackle harder topics such as good health versus bad health. There might be some hard truths in these chapters that you do not want to confront, but it is time to realize what your seemingly harmless bad habits might be doing to your body. Once you put those good and bad health habits behind you, we dive deep into dieting! I know, dieting can be a tricky and controversial subject. However, there are many studies that have shown how dieting contributes to your fertility and what you should and should not be doing to maximize your fertility.

Have you ever heard of natural birth control or family planning? Family planning does not necessarily have to involve hormonal contraceptives — that is the fallacy that we have been led to believe. Chapter seven tackles the topic of birth control. There are plenty of natural birth control methods that you can and should try before putting hormones into your body.

Chapters eight and nine circle back to some difficult topics. I will discuss the most well-known causes of miscarriages and the unfortunate reasons why miscarriages can happen to the most healthy women. It is never easy to confront the ghosts of our pasts or those concerns we have about the future. Everyone handles loss differently, but it is important to understand why the loss occurred and how you might prevent the loss from happening again. Chapter eight segues into chapter nine as we take on a definite focus on conceiving and how you can get pregnant. By the time you get into chapter nine, you should be more familiar with your body's hormones and your window of fertility, however, if you are not there yet, I will briefly recap how you can familiarize yourself with your body's most fertile time.

The ultimate goal of this guide is to help you carry a full-term and healthy pregnancy. You wanted to know how to get pregnant and how to do it safely and naturally while eliminating many of the risks that cause miscarriages. You now have all that information at your fingertips and stored in your brain. In chapter ten, I will go over what changes you can expect in your body when you begin expecting. I will also briefly reiterate the importance of diet and dietary changes you should make when you learn that you are expecting.

I hope that you go into this guide with a clean slate to absorb all of the information and that you come out with a far better understanding of your body and what it can do for you. Happy reading, good luck, and let's learn about our bodies!

Chapter 1: Fertility Awareness

You want to be aware of your own body. For a woman, fertility awareness is simply being conscious of your body's fertile and infertile phases during your menstrual cycle. While a lot of "don't ask, don't tell" exists around the functions of a woman's body, it has become time to change the narrative and education that women receive about their fertility.

Becoming aware of your menstrual cycle and what it means for your body is important on a multitude of levels. Not everyone who charts their monthly cycle is hoping to get pregnant — and this is where the beauty of being aware of your fertility lies. You can use this awareness to try and get pregnant, to avoid getting pregnant, and even as an overall checker of your health. Your menstrual cycle can tell you a lot about your body and your gynecological health, which can help you detect issues before they get worse.

There are no downsides to understanding your body on such a personal one on one level. When you begin to learn about your own fertility and you start becoming familiar with your body's responses during different phases of your cycle, you will become comfortable with terms such as basal body temperature, cervical positioning, and cervical mucus which are key factors to tracking your fertility. You will also start tracking how long each menstrual cycle lasts for you which will give you the answer to when your window of fertility is open. With fertility awareness, it only takes one small change and piece of knowledge to start a chain reaction toward further enlightenment about your menstrual health.

What Your Doctor Isn't Telling You About Fertility Awareness

So, if being aware of your fertility holds such benefits for women (primarily, knowing your own body and how to control it without hormonal supplements), then why are we still not told much about it? One might start to think that this is the teacher's job during those health classes in high school. Others might think it's a parent's job to teach their daughters about their bodies. Yet, we all get care at some point from our doctors and we still are not taught the basics of knowing our bodies. Why is this?

There are thousands of women in the world who struggle with their menstrual cycle, and they look to their doctors for help and advice. Often the only suggestion they are met with is a prescription for more hormonal contraceptives. We live in a day and age where irregular periods and unusual feminine bodily patterns are becoming more and more commonplace, yet the answers are not being taught. We have an entire generation of women who are uneducated about how they can best help themselves.

It can become easy to create an atmosphere of hostility between you and your doctor once you find out what they failed to teach you about your body. However, we must also understand that a majority of the doctors and other medical professionals that we come into contact with have never been taught about fertility awareness themselves. This is not to say that they are not aware of family planning methods but more so that their information is inaccurate or incomplete when it comes to the truth about fertility awareness.

Fertility is a tricky subject in the medical community, and not many professionals in the medical field are handed all the tools they need in school. It's a system that is set up to fail women.

There are a few things that your doctor might not know or might not tell you regarding your own fertility and being aware of your body. For example, you are often handed different hormone prescriptions at the doctors and sometimes it can take a while to find the right hormone dosage for you and your body. These hormones can either help you get pregnant, prevent pregnancy, or can be taken for a host of other "health benefits." However, what they often end up doing is messing with your internal menstrual cycle and changing the way that your body functions. It can be a tricky slope for doctors to navigate as they may either be uneducated about the benefits of fertility awareness or because they are caught in the middle of a billion-dollar industry that profits off of women taking hormone replacements.

However, the raw truth about fertility awareness and charting your cycle (the one that your doctor probably won't share with you) is that you will get a better understanding of how your reproductive system works. You will stop being the passenger in your feminine health and start taking back control of the steering wheel. A woman's issues don't always require pills or injections to solve, sometimes it is as simple as charting your own cycle.

Why Fertility Awareness Is Important

Now that you can understand the fine line your doctor walks on when it comes to talking to you about your reproductive health, you might still be wondering about the big deal regarding fertility awareness. It is important to note that while there are healthcare professionals who are ignorant about charting your cycle, there are also healthcare professionals who have dedicated their lives to educating other women about the benefits that charting will bring them.

Having basic knowledge of your fertility gives you an important tool to use in your arsenal of personal health. The benefits that you will get when you understand your fertility are that you will know when your body is fertile, when your body is infertile, how to tell if there is a more severe problem with your body, and why your body might be going through certain symptoms or changes.

Most women in the world between the ages of 13 to 50 experience a period. We have learned to associate this as a sign that we are not pregnant, but we don't know much more than that about our own menstrual cycles. Oddly enough, while women are familiar with the time of the month that they actively bleed, they often do not know that this is not the most significant part of your monthly cycle. In fact, menstruation is merely one part of an entire cycle. When it comes to your reproductive cycle, ovulation is the most vital phase, not menstruation. To find out when your body is ovulating (the stage where your body releases a mature egg in the hopes that it will be fertilized) you need to chart your cycle, as each woman's menstrual cycle will differ based on their own body's natural processes. You can typically expect ovulation to happen somewhere between 11 and 16 days before you begin to bleed (menstruate).

Your ovaries will go through different phases of life and health. This simply means that your ovaries have stages where they might secret hormones better during your younger years of life than they do in your later stages of life. The name of the concept that is most commonly associated with the lifespan of your ovaries and the ovarian cycle is the ovarian continuum (Vigil 2012). This continuum refers to the different types and levels of activity that your ovaries operate on as your reproductive life ages.

For a brief moment, let us assume that your purpose is to get pregnant. This can get costly and expensive when you are constantly buying testing kits to find out when your perfect window of fertility is. When you are aware of your menstrual cycle from day one to day 28 (or beyond depending on your menstrual cycle) you'll notice when you ovulate and when you don't. For example, you will be able to tell if your body fails to enter the ovulation phase during your monthly cycle. What does this mean for you? Several things, the first is that you know a mature egg has not been released that cycle. If your body skips out on the ovulation phase, you also become aware that there might be another issue with your body. This is because when a woman ovulates, it is a marker that she is in good health. When you are so familiar with your body, you can take a problem to your healthcare provider long before they will ever detect it. No one knows your body better than you do. No one has the potential to understand your body and your fertility better than you do.

This is why fertility awareness is important to women, it can mean the difference between good health and bad health. You put yourself in control of your own reproductive health and trust your body to tell you what it needs and what it might be missing.

A Path to Achieving True Reproductive Health

The bigger issue on your mind might be regarding your reproductive health. Let us say that you are becoming more familiar with your body and its phases and that you understand the importance of fertility awareness. How do you begin to use this information to achieve true reproductive health? How can it best benefit you in your journey to conceive?

Your reproductive health involves more than your uterus. When I refer to your reproductive health in this guide, I am talking about you and your body being in a state of well-being and health mentally, physically, and socially. You can have no diseases or illnesses to worry about but there might still be snags in your journey to reproductive health if any function — such as your mental state — has a glitch to it. When you obtain true reproductive health as a woman, you are able to partake in a safe sexual lifestyle and reproduce with your partners if you chose to do so. This means that you have the ability to get pregnant when you want to based on your window of opportunity (fertility).

Where do you begin to take care of your reproductive health? Women in today's society are not taught how to care for their mental and physical well-being, especially as it relates to their reproductive processes.

The first thing you should do when taking an active role in your reproductive health is to choose your method of birth control or family planning wisely. This is an extremely important decision and a very personal one as well. When you decide to take birth control and add a foreign level of a hormone to your body's natural cycles, it can cause damaging side effects. This is where you should not be afraid to have open and honest conversations with your doctors. Do not let them simply prescribe a birth control pill to you, but rather educate yourself about the birth control they are suggesting and find out what your other options might be.

Women around the world suffer from the drastic side effects of birth control. Side effects could include a lower libido which affects your reproductive health. You could also experience extreme mood swings, a sudden loss or gain of weight, or a change in your acne or even bodily secretions. There was a study conducted in 2019 by a research group studying obstetrics and gynecology that encompassed over 7,000 Polish women who ranged from ages 18 to 35. It studied the effects that birth control had on these women, and the most common side effects experienced were a lowered libido, with 39 percent of the women experiencing a significantly lower sexual drive. An additional 22 percent of the women found that they gained weight while on the contraceptives (Int J Environ Res Public Health 2019).

This is not the only study that has been conducted regarding the reproductive health of women. A Dutch study that was published in 2014 also indicated that women who had taken oral contraceptives struggled with understanding and recognizing emotions that were displayed via facial expression — in short, their emotional intelligence was affected (Eur Neuropsychopharmacol 2014). While there are birth control methods that are available without hormones, you might want to look at the Fertility Awareness Method. You can also double up on this method by using condoms. With the FAM (Fertility Awareness Method) you track your cycle through your basal body temperature, cervical mucus, and your monthly calendar. There are many ways to chart out your cycle, however, the main goal is to locate the times of your cycle where you will be fertile and infertile. If you are avoiding getting pregnant, then you will simply either abstain or use condoms during your fertile period.

When you are taking into consideration your reproductive health, you want to make sure that you are practicing safe sex. This might seem benign to you, but the lack of stress and worry on both your mental and physical systems is an important part of your reproductive health. Remember that finding a method of family planning that works for you does not necessarily protect you from sexually transmitted infections (STI).

Make sure that any sexual partner is willing to partake in a conversation about sexual history — before you have sex. This is important because you want to make sure that they don't have infections they can pass to you, and you want to be honest about any infections you may or may not have had in the past. Condoms are one of the most common methods used to protect against STI's, so please use them. Particularly if you are not in a monogamous sexual situation. Remember that condoms also won't protect you against HPV (there is a vaccination for this that young women should get to aid in the protection against cervical cancer and genital warts). Be open and honest with your partner and make sure that they are trustworthy regarding their own sexual history. Don't stress over STI's when you know you can practice safe sex.

It goes without saying that my third point in this guide to your reproductive health is to get familiar with your cycle and track it! I promise you that this will be revolutionary in how you see your health. At the risk of sounding like a broken record (and I promise you this point will come back up throughout this guide) please track your cycle. You will be connected to your body, and you will also feel in control of your body. For example, those bizarre emotions that you experience throughout the month will suddenly make sense to you as you begin to track your cycle, and you will find ways to deal with them in healthier manners than before. If you were trying to make progress with your skin and possible issues with acne, tracking your cycle can be the most beneficial tool for you. This is not only about trying to track when you are fertile or infertile (though this is a great benefit!) but also about being an overall encompassing tool to your reproductive health.

You can track your cycle both manually on a physical calendar or you can use any one of the many apps that exist to help women chart their cycles.

You will need to keep up with drinking water. I know that everyone tells you about the importance of drinking water, but for a woman, it can affect more than your level of hydration. For example, if you become overly dehydrated then you can suffer from vaginal dryness which not only promotes discomfort during sexual intercourse but will also increase the likelihood of you suffering from a yeast infection. No one wants that, so do yourself a favor and drink your water every day!

If you find that you suffer from vaginal dryness during sexual intercourse, this could cause a distressing situation, particularly if the problem is ongoing. Vaginal dryness can happen for a multitude of reasons such as a lack of arousal, menopause, medication you might be taking, and even stress. Using additional lubrication can make intercourse more enjoyable for you.

Nothing is better for your reproductive health than making sure that both you and your doctor are aware of where you lie with your health. Make sure that you get your annual exams done by your doctor and don't be shy about checking yourself out as well. This includes examining your breasts to make sure they are healthy too. Remember that reproductive health does not mean only your uterus and vaginal areas. Your whole body needs to be healthy for full and true reproductive health. You will also learn the best times to examine your body once you get used to tracking your cycle and what your hormones do to change your body.

I know that periods can be an exhausting time for you, but they don't have to be particularly difficult. Pain and exhaustion are the most common symptoms women experience as they go through their menstruation phase. However, there are things that you can do in order to promote happy vibes during your menstruation. One of the best things that I can recommend is to find a menstruation product that works for you. Tampons might be your method of choice, but keep menstrual cups in mind too! There are a lot of revolutionary menstrual cup products that change the way women handle their flow.

Keep some time set aside for yourself during the week that you are menstruating. Don't overextend yourself and give all of your energy to other people. Giving yourself even a simple thirty minutes a day can significantly lessen the stress on your body and mind.

Women are susceptible to so many toxins in this life that affect our reproductive systems. There are toxins in the foods that we eat and the products that we use on and around our bodies. Make a concerted effort to avoid these toxins — particularly if you want children one day. I will go more in-depth about the toxins in your diet and what foods to avoid to boost your reproductive health.

Brief Recap

I know that each chapter might be packed with a lot of information to take in and absorb. This will be true particularly when we get to the meatier parts of this guide. In order to make sure that the bigger topics (and some of the smaller topics) stay fresh in your mind as you close out each chapter, I will take you through some of the main points that were covered.

- Your menstrual cycle involves more than your menstruation. Your menstruation is an important part of your monthly cycle, but ovulation is one of the most important parts as well. Ovulation is the phase where your body releases a mature egg. This happens normally 11 to 16 days before your menstruation begins.

- Your reproductive health involves more than your uterus and vaginal area and includes your overall mental and emotional health.

- There are toxins in the foods that we eat that impact our reproductive health.

- Many doctors are not educated about fertility awareness and are therefore at a disadvantage to teach their female patients how to track their cycles and the changes in their bodies.

- Keeping track of your menstrual cycle can help you find your fertile and infertile times of the month. It can also help you identify if there is an abnormality in your body that is new or that has newly come to your attention.

- Your fertility awareness is your best tool and form of personal protection.

Chapter 2: What Is Your "Cycle?"

As we delve into chapter two, you will experience both new and old information. If you come across a section of information that you are already familiar with, be patient and add it to your active memory. Keep it fresh in your mind as you read because all of the information ties in together to give you a bigger picture.

It is important to be aware of your reproductive organs, your menstrual cycle, and the reproductive process. The reason for this is that it all ties into the fertility awareness issue. Getting pregnant involves each one of these sections, and having an understanding of it will help you streamline your journey into changing the way you naturally family plan.

A Quick Lesson on Reproductive Anatomy

Producing more offspring is the purpose of reproduction (at least, normally this is the end result). While your reproductive system makes you uniquely qualified to carry on the next generation of the human population, it is not a necessary feature of life. This means that your reproductive system is not vital to your life like your heart or lungs. However, many women find great joy in producing offspring and many want to.

When it comes to reproduction, two important sex cells are fundamental to the process. These sex cells, called gametes, come in two forms — male and female. Their first meeting point occurs in the reproductive system of the female. This is where your egg will have been released and awaits fertilization by the male gamete (sperm).

While both the male and female reproductive systems are needed to reproduce, the hosting of the zygote (fertilized egg) occurs in the female reproductive system. So, what exactly is the female reproductive system composed of? You might think you are familiar with your own reproductive organs, but there are a surprising number of women who are misinformed about their own bodies.

Let us begin with the vulva. This is the external part that begins the female reproductive organs. "Vulva" simply means covering, which is apt since it covers and protects the opening of the vaginal canal. It also protects other organs of your body.

Your mons pubis is the area of flesh that you find right on top of your vaginal opening. Your labia are the fleshy flaps of skin that surround the vaginal opening. Labia means lips, and so these are often called the lips of the vagina. Around the front of your vulva, you will find a small organ called the clitoris. It has thousands of nerve endings and is right in the center of were the labia folds join together. Your urethra is located below the clitoris and between the labia. This is the channel that will transport pee from inside your bladder to the outside. Many people think that you pee out of the main opening in your labia, but this is not true. Your urethra has this job.

The vagina, uterus, ovaries, and the fallopian tubes make up a woman's internal reproductive organs. Your vagina is essentially a muscle. It is tubelike and hollow, extending from the opening of the vagina to the uterus. Since the vagina has muscular walls that form the tube, it is able to expand and contract as necessary. This muscular tube is the reason your vagina is able to hold onto your slim tampons or other menstrual cups and also accommodate the birth of a baby. However, the tube is not just muscular and dry but covered in mucous membranes which keeps the area moist and keeps bad bacteria out.

So, why do women have a vagina? The obvious purpose of the vagina is to assist in sexual intercourse. However, the vagina does more than merely serve as a conduit for sex. The vagina becomes the canal through which the baby will travel out of your body. It is also the area where blood from your menstrual phase will exit your body.

There is a thin lining of tissue that covers part of the vaginal opening known as the hymen. Each female has her own unique hymen and it is typically associated with being broken during a woman's first time having intercourse. While this may be true, the hymen can also break in many other ways throughout a woman's life. When it is stretched or ripped, it can bleed and cause some slight discomfort at the moment.

As you know, the baby comes down through the birth canal and out of the vaginal opening. Connected to the vaginal canal is the uterus. Your uterus (also called the womb) is connected right around an area called the cervix. You might have heard your doctor refer to your cervix. It can be considered the neck of the womb and is comprised of walls that are thick. The cervix is the reason your menstrual cups don't get lost inside your uterus. The opening to the cervix is small and controlled (picture a straw opening) so it will not open wide enough to allow passage for a menstrual device. This is why labor during childbirth can take a long time because the cervix has to expand wide enough to accommodate the size of the baby.

When you think of the shape of your womb, picture a pear and turn it upside down. Then add some lining around the pear and a few muscular walls and bam! There is your uterus. Have you ever heard that the tongue is one of the strongest muscles in the human body? Well, the uterus houses some of the strongest muscles in the female body. Not only do these muscles work for a woman on an everyday basis, but they expand, contract, and move in order to fit a growing baby. They also push when it is time for that baby to come out.

Keep picturing your upside-down pear. At the very top of the uterus, you will find tubes at the corners that serve as the connection between the ovaries and uterus. These connecting tubes are the fallopian tubes. Your ovaries will be found on the upper part of your uterus to the left and to the right. They are oval in shape. This is where your eggs are created, stored, and released at the right time of your cycle. As ovulation occurs, your ovary will send an egg down the fallopian tube into your uterus (do you see how all the information is slowly tying together?) Your ovaries have an important role to play in your body since they are also responsible for your hormones, estrogen and progesterone.

Your entire reproductive system works together to create a baby and push that same baby out when the time is right. It has a multitude of jobs and none are related to your breathing or your heart beating. Isn't it incredible that your body contains this entire set of organs and processes that exist solely for sexual reproduction and intercourse? And at the same time, it serves as the house for the unborn baby? Amazing!

Ovulation is going to come up quite often, particularly as I go more in-depth about this phase of your menstrual cycle when you begin learning about charting your cycle. As your ovaries send an egg down your fallopian tube and into your uterus, it begins to patiently wait for fertilization. When that does not happen, normally after a period of two weeks, your body will shed the egg and you will menstruate. As we delve deeper into the topic of your cycle, we will also cover premenstrual syndrome, commonly referred to as PMS. PMS affects a woman's body in many ways before their periods begin. It can include acne, fatigue, bloating, aches and pains in the body, constipation, and even headaches. You are also most likely familiar with cramping which commonly occurs during a woman's menstruation.

If you are charting your cycle and you have sex during your window of fertility then fertilization of your egg might occur. This means that you won't enter the menstruation phase of your cycle, but rather, the male's sperm will fertilize the egg. Within 5 days, that fertilized egg will become a blastocyst (essentially a sac of cells filled with fluid). Implantation will then occur and the stages of development will progress until a baby is born.

Your reproductive anatomy is vital to the birthing process, and it will all work together to produce the baby that you have long-awaited. So, what exactly is your menstrual cycle?

Your Menstrual Cycle

I can tell you what your menstrual cycle is not — it is not simply the week that you bleed. Your menstrual cycle occurs in four different phases, and it can normally take a month to cycle back to stage or phase one. The reason for your menstrual cycle is because your reproductive system goes through certain processes every month that are a direct result of the hormones released in your body. For example, the estrogen and progesterone that your ovaries release into your body are part of a chain of events that prompt other phases to begin.

Most women do not realize that your menstrual cycle actually begins with menstruation. This is not the end of your cycle, but the very first part. The first day that your period begins (the first day of bleeding) is day one of your menstrual phase. Stage one is called the "menstrual phase." This phase can last anywhere from three to a total of seven days, it depends on each woman's body and its processes. As you go through the menstrual phase, you will shed a total average of one-quarter of a cup of blood.

The second stage of your menstrual cycle will be the "follicular phase." This is the stage your body uses to start preparing to get pregnant. The estrogen hormone that is released in your body will signal to your uterine lining that it needs to thicken and prepare for an egg to be fertilized. Your ovarian follicles will begin to grow as well during this phase as your follicle-stimulating hormone (FSH) kicks into gear. Your hormones really come alive as they get the womb ready for a baby. The follicles that grow hold onto the eggs, but only one of these eggs will normally be selected to be the one that is held as an option for fertilization. Estrogen continues to be on the rise, and as you get ready to ovulate, your estrogen levels will be at an all-time high.

The "ovulation phase" is the third stage of your menstrual cycle. Many women have a regular cycle that lasts 28 days. If you experience a 28-day cycle, then your ovulation normally happens as you enter day 14 of the cycle. Remember that right before you started this third phase of your cycle, your estrogen was at an all-time high, this causes another hormone called luteinizing hormone (LH) to gear into action. This new hormone makes the ovarian follicle let go of the egg that it has been holding on to and the egg then travels towards the fallopian tube and down into the uterus. Because menstrual cycle lengths can vary, ovulation might happen anywhere between 11 and 16 days from the day you actually begin your cycle over again. During ovulation, your mature egg will travel towards your uterus in the hopes that it gets fertilized. This takes a few days, and while the egg is moving along the fallopian tube, your uterine lining will continue to thicken. After 3 or 4 days, your egg will find itself in the uterus. You have around 24 hours before the egg gets frustrated and starts to fade.

The "luteal phase" starts as ovulation is complete and your egg starts to degenerate. This is the fourth and final stage of your menstrual cycle before it starts all over again. The follicle that is now no longer has an egg becomes what is known as a corpus luteum. The cells of this create more estrogen and also turn up the production of progesterone. Progesterone is the hormone that prompts your uterine lining to get ready for the fertilized egg.

During the luteal phase, you can get pregnant if you have unprotected sex. Once the egg is fertilized, it will attach to your uterine lining. However, in the absence of a fertilized egg, the uterine lining will begin to shed and you will find yourself back at day one of the menstrual phase and your body will go through each phase again on a loop.

The Reproductive Process

Understanding the phases of your menstrual cycle is easy

because they are so straightforward. You might even begin to recognize once your body shifts into each phase. As you deal with menstruation, often it becomes rather easy and natural to understand the different cycles and the process of bleeding. What about when an egg is fertilized in the womb? How does a baby grow? These are all things you would want to know as you prepare to become a potential mother.

You already know that when reproduction starts, a female egg is in the uterus and it gets fertilized by sperm. The fertilized egg is called a zygote. This moment in time is commonly called conception. However, you are not pregnant until this egg that is fertilized implants itself within the uterine lining — this is why your hormones were thickening your uterine lining.

Both the sperm cell and the female egg are necessary for procreation as they contain the codes and DNA that are necessary for reproduction. As the two cells merge into one, they go from each carrying 23 chromosomes to a combined 46 chromosomes. The fertilized egg eventually divides itself into a blastocyst which buries itself into the thickened uterine lining and prepares to develop. The blastocyst does not reach the uterine lining instantly, and it can take about five days before the fertilized egg is implanted. As it implants, more changes and developments occur within the cell. On day 15 (this means the 15th day since conception began, not since sexual intercourse) the blastocyst changes into an embryonic disc. The cells begin to develop support structures that will later become vital parts of the developing baby. For example, the yolk sac that develops in an area of the embryonic disc will later develop into the digestive tract of the baby. Across from the yolk sac, the amnion will fill up with the fluid that the embryo will float in as it develops.

There are common misconceptions about when your baby becomes a fetus. This does not happen at the moment of conception as it takes time for the cells to grow and develop into a growing baby. As you now know, on day 15 the embryonic disc forms, and this starts what is known as the embryonic period. During this period, the embryonic disc is flat in structure and develops itself into three different layers. These layers are the ectoderm, the endoderm, and the mesoderm. Each different layer will be responsible for the development of organs that are vital to human function. The layers will develop and curve like a banana until they slowly form the shape of a body.

In week 4, after conception, the embryo will develop its head and a tail. Its heart is also developed during this week and it will begin beating on its own. In the six weeks following week 4, the embryo will begin to grow and develop distinct human features such as eyes, limbs that form the arms and legs, areas of the brain, and the vertebrae of the spine. Week 10 is when the embryo is now considered a fetus. This means that by week 10, a developing baby will have all of its basic human physical traits.

It is important to remember that when doctors and other professionals refer to pregnancy and weeks, they measure it in gestational age. This means the measurement of weeks it taking place from the woman's very first day of her last period. It can also be measured in age by its fetal/embryonic age which is merely its actual age from the day of conception. For the purposes of this chapter, we will be basing the timeline off of the gestational age.

You often need to wait a few months before you find out the sex of your baby, however, this has already begun to form by the time the baby is at week 6 of development. The necessary reproductive genes act in the embryonic stage and the embryo will have gonads and its genitalia.

The sperm is the deciding factor on whether the child is a boy or girl. Since the female egg will have an X chromosome. The male sperm will deliver either an X chromosome or a Y chromosome. The resulting pairing of these chromosomes determines the sex. For example, an XY pair will prompt the gonads to start developing into testes during week 7 of development and you will be growing a boy. If it is an XX pair, then the gonads that are developed in week 6 will turn into ovaries around week 8 and you will be growing a girl. For the males, their testes will start producing the testosterone hormone and this prompts the male genitalia to begin forming at week 10. If this hormone is lacking, female genitalia will form instead.

You now have a fetus that is growing with its own beating heart inside the uterus at week 10 of your pregnancy. The fetus is able to continue to develop and grow because the umbilical cord that is attached to the fetus feeds it blood that is packed with the necessary nutrients for its survival. The placenta has an important job while the fetus is developing in your womb. It needs to ensure that the growing baby gets oxygen and nutrients, but also that all waste and toxins are removed. The baby will continue to advance and grow as it is getting those nutrients, forming the necessary bones and muscles. The skin and other connecting tissues will also form at this stage in the womb. The baby's organ systems will begin to kick in and start working in a rudimentary way.

By the time the baby grows to week 36, it should have all basic human components and organs. The finer features are developed and the baby's facial features and other body parts will have their own unique properties. In week 36, you can expect that labor might begin. The first step in labor is for you to begin to dilate. This simply means that the hormones in your body (you really will have a lot of hormones at this stage!) will signal that your uterine walls should start contracting. When you are in labor, your cervix will continue to dilate (normally, you want to be dilated at 10cm for the baby to fit through) and your contractions will guide the baby out the birthing canal. Your contractions might be intense as they need to be strong enough to expel the baby from the uterus through the cervix and out of the vaginal opening. At this stage, your baby has been born. The final steps of labor involve a few more contractions so that the placenta is pushed out as well.

Brief Recap

This chapter contained a lot of information regarding reproduction and the menstrual cycle. Some of it may have been old but refreshed in your mind, and other bits of information might have been entirely new and changed your view on these processes.

- Your menstrual cycle has four stages, the menstrual phase, the follicular phase, the ovulation phase, and the luteal phase.

- Your menstrual cycle begins on the first day of your period.

- Reproductive anatomy is not vital to the survival of a woman but is necessary in order to reproduce and conceive.

- A woman's hormones during her menstrual cycle will signal the uterine lining to thicken in preparation for a fertilized egg to implant. This thickened lining sheds and is passed during the period if the egg goes unfertilized.

- At week 4, your baby's heart is formed and will start beating. By 10 weeks, your embryo is considered a fetus and has rudimentarily developed and formed.

- The male sperm cell will deliver the X or Y sex chromosome that determines the baby's sex.

Chapter 3: Charting Your Cycle

Welcome to the beginning of change! I hope that you are able to learn how to chart your cycle and that you implement the changes in your life. There is knowledge and power that lies in charting your own cycle, and you begin to control your own body.

Doesn't that sound like a dream? For a change, instead of letting the doctors guide you about your own body, you will be in control. You will know what you need to give your body and the reasons behind certain changes in your body. You will also be able to know first if something is wrong and bring it up with your healthcare provider. In short, you will have full body autonomy and freedom.

You can chart in more than one way, and I will cover all the necessary basics that are important to understand when beginning your charting journey. Keep in mind as you go through this chapter that there might be an adjustment process or a learning curve. Allow yourself the space and the time to get used to charting your cycle and develop that familiarity with your body. You can keep up a simple menstrual calendar, a specific fertility chart, and even both if you choose. It is up to you what level of charting you want to do. If you are trying to conceive, then I recommend that you keep a specific fertility awareness chart so that you can track your most fertile days of the month.

Why and How Should I Chart?

You should chart because it empowers you to become your body's own advocate. There will be no authority other than your own that has complete and total control over your health.

You can chart in many different ways. If you are only charting when you bleed (the menstrual phase of your cycle) then you can use any calendar you choose. It can be an online calendar, the one on your phone, a paper calendar, a period tracker app calendar, or any other type of calendar. If you would rather have a more structured calendar, there are many options online for you to download with specific menstrual information.

The main goal of charting your cycle is for you to note down when you are bleeding, any vaginal secretions, physical changes, and any emotional changes you go through or feel. Encompassed in the physical changes that you will chart are your pain levels if you experience cramping, how heavy your flow is from one day to the next, alternatively how light your flow of bleeding is from one day to the next, if your libido increases or decreases, and your energy levels. Do you see what I mean about getting up close and personal with your body? You will also chart your breasts and whether they get swollen, are they tender, do they feel firmer? Any change that you think is vital or necessary to chart, go ahead and chart it. This is how you get to know your body.

You might have already heard about the Fertility Awareness Method (FAM). I have briefly mentioned it in the chapters above, and if this is your first time hearing about FAM, don't worry about it. This method is not complicated at all, it only takes a minute to wrap your head around the necessary steps and things to keep track of.

This is not the only method you can use to track your cycle, but it is one of the easiest and most commonly used methods. The reason that FAM is so popular is that it helps you with both tracking your gynecological health also with natural family planning and fertility tracking for pregnancy.

When you get into FAM and start tracking your body's changes, you will have to become more vigilant about the changes in your cervical fluid. You will also start tracking any color changes, size changes, and the shape of your cervix. This is because the cervix is one of your best friends when tracking your fertility.

The Fertility Awareness Method is based on science and uses scientific principles to work as the best tool for understanding your body. While you know that you have four stages of your menstrual cycle, it can be split into three main stages. These stages are:

1. The pre-ovulatory infertile phase

2. The fertile phase.

3. The post-ovulatory infertile phase.

You can guess by the prefixes of each phase where each one ends and begins. Ovulation still remains at the center of these stages. I will get into your fertility signs later on in this chapter, but for now, you need to know that you will use those signs to determine what phase of fertility you are in. The main fertility signs you will familiarize yourself with are your basal body temperature, your cervical fluid, and your cervical position.

Thanks to estrogen and progesterone — the two main hormones controlling and influencing your menstrual cycles — your body drops hints all day long about what these hormones are doing to your body. Sometimes they like to wreak havoc on your systems!

Estrogen is the main event in your body as this hormone takes total control of the very first half of your menstrual cycle. Progesterone doesn't like to get left behind, and it comes out in the latter half of your cycle to dominate over estrogen. Your luteinizing hormone (LH) plays an important role in your cycle as this is the hormone that kicks the egg from the ovaries. When you buy a testing kit to check for ovulation, they merely measure the amount of LH in your body. Do you see how this could easily be kept track of on your own so you could save yourself the expensive pee tests?

In each cycle that you have, you will only ovulate once. Normally only one egg is released during ovulation, but there are some circumstances of two eggs being released (hence, fraternal twins exist). The egg will last for roughly 12-24 hours in the uterus awaiting fertilization. It is important to know and be aware of all of this because charting that period of fertility really does come down to precise days when you are trying to conceive.

The good news is that you don't have to have sex the day you ovulate or are most fertile to increase your chances of getting pregnant because sperm lasts more than 24 hours. In an environment where the cervical fluid is at its most fertile, sperm will last for around 5 days. In less than fertile conditions, sperm will survive for around 2 days.

Important Signs of Fertility

There are two different types of fertility signs. Primary fertility signs and secondary fertility signs. I have already mentioned the primary fertility signs, but I am going to go more in-depth with their explanations now so that you understand their importance and how to chart them.

Basal Body Temperature (BBT)

Your Basal Body Temperature is also commonly called your Waking Temperature. Yes, this means you will be taking your temperature as you wake up every morning — a small step to add to your morning routine that will make all the difference to understanding your body.

In the early mornings, you will want to record what your temperature is to get an accurate summation of your ovulation phases. Before ovulation occurs, your temperatures will be around 97°F and 97.5°F (alternatively 36.11°C and 36.38°C). After ovulation occurs, your basal body temperature will rise between 97.6°F and 98.6°F (36.44°C and 37°C). For the most accurate and precise readings, use a digital thermometer. You can also invest in a basal thermometer that is designed specifically for tracking your BBT. This is because the changes in body temperatures can be so minuscule a regular thermometer might give you errors in your readings.

Once ovulation is complete, your body temperature will continue to stay up. It will only begin to lower again when you enter the phase to start your menstrual cycle over again. However, if during your phase of fertility you do get pregnant then you will see your BBT stay high for a period of more than 18 days.

As you test yourself and get comfortable with what normal temperatures are for you and your body, you will understand your personal temperature pattern. You will know what is normal for you before you ovulate and when your temperature changes to indicate that you are ovulating. Charting these changes comes in handy because you get an overall picture of your average BBT over a couple of days. This lessens the likelihood of error if you were only thinking of your day to day temperature. You need to allow yourself to view the bigger picture so you can accurately pinpoint your period of fertility.

If you see an increase today but a decrease tomorrow, that can be a discrepancy that leaves you with inaccurate information about your body. However, if you see that over the last two days your BBT raised and stayed up then you will know that your ovulation has started.

BBT testing does have a downfall: you only find out about ovulation after it has started and not before. If you want an accurate picture of your ovulation before it happens you need to pay attention to your cervical fluid and position. It takes time to see the cohesion between the three primary fertility signs, however, if you accurately chart out your cycle for a minimum of three cycles, you will begin to see them interacting with one another. They exist in their own circle as well.

Everyone's body is different. This is true for all women. While there is an average to base measurements off of, please remember that this does not accurately represent the billions of women in the world. This is why I advocate that you chart because that is how you will get to know what is normal and right for your body. A guide can only go so far until you put in your personal work.

Keep in mind that there are things that will affect your BBT and cause you to have an inaccurate reading for your FAM. For example:

- If you have a fever.
- If you have had a lack of sleep the night before. You want to have more than four hours of sleep for an accurate reading.
- Drinking alcohol the previous night.
- If you eat or drink before you take your temperature (this is mainly if you take your temperature via oral means).
- If you are not consistent with the times that you take your temperature.
- Possible thyroid issues.
- If you heated your body using a heating pad or blanket.

Cervical Fluid

Finally! The fluid that I have talked so much about. Your cervical fluid is the secretion that you produce around the time you begin to ovulate. This secretion is what lets the sperm cells reach your freshly dropped egg. You can liken it to seminal fluid, except that it is in strict relation to the female genetic makeup. However, both seminal fluid and cervical fluid have similar duties. The cervical fluid you have will also protect sperm and give it a chance to reach your egg, it does this by serving as an alkaline substance in your acidic vagina. The acid in your vagina's pH level would normally kill the sperm off. Your cervical fluid is present to protect the sperm that could potentially father a future baby for you. Consider it as a guard dog. I say this because your cervical fluid helps nourish the sperm as it travels to your egg. It also filters out what can and cannot enter your personal chambers. One of the more important jobs that your cervical fluid does to assist you in getting pregnant is that it helps the sperm take its head off so that it is ready to fertilize the egg once it breaks into it. In short, your cervical fluid wants you to get pregnant.

How does your cervical fluid tell you when you are ovulating? Thanks to the indicators from your estrogen hormone, your cervical fluid will begin to appear more liquid in consistency as ovulation gets closer. As you finish your period, you should be on the lookout to chart your cervical fluid. For example, you will probably see it a few days after your period finishes. Your cervical fluid should take the shape of a sticky and creamy secretion to a clearer secretion that is slippery to the touch. You might also find that it is stretchy almost like taffy stretches as you observe it. When your estrogen reaches its highest limit and then drops back down to lower levels, your cervical fluid will disappear. This happens in a matter of hours due to the drastic hormone change. Your progesterone takes over at this point in the ovulation phase. You likely won't see your cervical fluid in such a consistency again. Until the cycle starts over.

Okay, I know right now you might be weirded out by inspecting your own cervical fluid. Remember though, this is your body. There is nothing shameful in understanding your body. One of the best ways to track your cervical fluid is to use your finger and run it over your vaginal lips. However, if you do not feel comfortable doing that yet, you can also use some tissue. The point of this is to identify the consistency of the cervical fluid. It might take some getting used to at first, but soon when you do this you will ask the questions in your mind almost as if it were second nature. Does it feel dry when you wipe or smooth? Does it easily glide over your vaginal lips or is there resistance? You already guessed it, but when your cervical fluid dries up, the tissue won't glide smoothly over your lips. The closer you get to ovulation, you will find that the tissue starts gliding easily over your lips because your cervical fluid gets wetter.

There is an entire list of things that can affect your cervical fluid's consistency similar to the list of things that affect your BBT. The issues that may impact your cervical fluid are:

- Lubricants used for intercourse
- Spermicides used as protection against pregnancy
- Vaginal infections
- Semen
- Antihistamines (these usually dry out your cervical fluid)

Hormonal birth control can also affect your cervical fluid. For example, stopping birth control can impact your cervical fluid by either stopping your production of it temporarily or creating a creamy consistency in your cervical fluid that lasts months after you have stopped the birth control. It is important to keep an eye out for all of these different factors as you begin charting the consistency and appearance of your cervical fluid every day.

Cervical Position

Your cervix is another main giveaway when you are tracking your ovulation through natural family planning. It changes as you progress through your menstrual cycle. Sometimes the change is easy to detect, other times you have to pay a little bit more attention to your cervix. You need to practice getting comfortable with your body because one of the easiest ways to check the change in your cervix (especially at certain times during your cycle) is to use your middle or index finger and feel the shape of your cervix.

Normally, when you inspect your cervix it will be firm. The closer you get to ovulation, your cervix will get softer and easier to press against. You will also find as you familiarize yourself with your cervix that it can be felt lower in your vagina and it stays closed. However, as estrogen and progesterone send their signals during your cycle, you will find that your cervix will rise higher and open up around ovulation.

Your cervix gives away a lot when it comes to ovulation. Not only will you see the difference in it being firm or soft and closed or open, but you will also notice its angle and position change. Right as ovulation occurs, your cervix moves to become straighter rather than angled.

Secondary Signs of Fertility

You might recall that I mentioned you have your three primary signs of fertility to chart: basal body temperature, cervical fluid, and cervical position. You can chart or simply look out for these secondary signs that indicate you are ovulating. I personally find it is easier to chart them, especially since this helps keep you in the habit of charting.

- You might feel an ache or symptom of pain near one of your ovaries.

- Your libido could increase.

- You could feel bloated.

Not everyone experiences these secondary fertility signs, or you might experience them for one month and then not the next. However, they are still good indicators to look out for when trying to track the fertile phase of your cycle. Use all the tools at your disposal so that your charting is at its most accurate.

Charting Those Fertility Signs

Charting your fertility can be really simple. Essentially you pay attention to your body's signs and you record the data that you find. There will be some daily active work needed but none of it will take you more than a minute or two.

For the more tech-savvy population, there are a host of mobile applications that you can use to help you track the fertile and infertile periods of your cycle. I personally love the calendar tracking method. I use a diary with a daily calendar where I can track what goes on with my body. Alternatively, there are a plethora of fertility trackers available for free online, you can download one of those templates if it helps you.

You know by now that there are so many good things that you can track while charting your body's phases. The main one is obviously that you are in your fertile period and your hormones are functioning as they should. Charting is so important because it can help you detect both those good signs that you want to see, but it can also help you find a bad sign before it progresses into something worse.

For example, if you skip out on your ovulation phase one cycle you might realize that there is a deeper issue going on and that will prompt you to see your doctor. You can also discover when you are feeling under the weather and combat feelings of illness early on. This is because you are paying attention to your body and being finely aware of little changes such as temperature changes.

Brief Recap

Charting will make all the difference to the way that you live, and contrary to what the general public makes it out to be, charting is super easy! Here are some key ideas to remember when you begin charting:

- Don't overwhelm yourself. Take it slow and easy. Start out with the calendar method. This is normally an easy and simple way to track your changes. Applications can have so many aspects to them that it can be confusing for someone who is recently learning about their body. As you feel more comfortable with tracking your cycle, then you should move to an application on your phone if that is more convenient.

- Take yourself out on dates and break down that barrier of shyness or embarrassment that you share with your own body. Try and do one thing every day that brings you out of your comfort zone and makes you feel better about your body.

- Your basal body temperature can easily be tracked every day with a digital thermometer for the most accurate reading.

- Your cervical fluid will be stretchy and slippery when you are ovulating, but dry when you are not.

- Your cervix changes position and becomes soft when you are ovulating.

- Charting your period can help you keep track of all the healthy signs in your body, but it can also help you detect if you might be sick or if there is an issue you need to bring to your doctor's attention.

Chapter 4: What Bad Health Means for Fertility

There is a key difference between good health and bad health, and while you might feel like you are in good health, you might be participating in unhealthy behaviors that affect your fertility. No one wants to be told that the choices they are making are directly affecting their fertility but sometimes the truth is hard to swallow.

Bad health can negatively affect your fertility in more ways than just one. Take a deep breath before carrying on with this chapter. I know it might seem scary right now, and you might want to close this guide out of fear, but you can do this. My aim is not to scare you, but to educate you. Our healthcare system has failed many women when it comes to educating us about our bodies, and it is high time we take back the power over our bodies.

I want to take a serious moment to discuss the issues that plague women and their bodies when it comes to issues with fertility. They affect us on so many levels and many times, the issues might be preventable if we knew the correct help to seek or methods to employ. Remember, bad health can often be turned around with some simple changes. It isn't the end of the world, and you can always find avenues for support.

Irregular Cycles and Anovulation

Normally, the menstrual cycle takes 28 days to complete and

start over again. This number does vary from woman to woman with some cycles being shorter and other cycles being longer. Irregular menstrual cycles are more common than you might think. However, don't freak out yet. There is some wiggle room if your menstrual cycle takes longer than 28 days to complete (you will know exactly how many days it takes you when you start charting your cycles). Any cycle that takes longer than 35 days to complete is considered an irregular cycle. This is also true if the length of your cycle tends to vary — this means that one month your cycle is 21 days and the next it is 38 days. Varied cycles are considered irregular because, by the time you finish puberty, your menstrual cycle should be established in a routine.

Generally, a woman's period starts when she is a young girl anywhere from the ages of 11 to 16 years of age. A woman's menstrual cycle won't stop until she reaches menopause — that is if everything is working as it should be.

You might hear irregular menstrual cycles referred to as oligomenorrhea, or alternatively as irregular periods. The term, period, is often used because women normally only mark the times of the month that they are actively bleeding as their period and not the entire menstrual cycle. Keep in mind that it is not always bad health that causes an irregular period, and you must be aware of all factors that could impact your menstrual cycle. For example, if you change your birth control methods from one pill to another or to an implant over a patch then that creates a hormonal shift in your body. This will change how frequently or how regularly you get your period until your body normalizes under the new birth control. Menopause and workouts like endurance exercises can also affect your hormone balance and as a result, impact your menstrual cycle.

So, what do you do if you get irregular menstrual cycles but you are nowhere near the age for menopause and you haven't switched your method of contraception recently? There are steps you can take to seek out advice and help regarding irregular menstrual cycles that occur during your formative reproductive years. Narrowing down the causes for an irregular cycle is the first thing you should do.

Hormonal imbalance is often the first cause that gets checked in regards to irregular cycles, they are also normally the main culprit. Estrogen and progesterone are both needed to help regulate menstrual cycles, and when one overproduces or does not produce enough, problems can occur. Keep in mind when you suspect hormones that there are hormonal issues that you are not going through a hormonal event such as menopause, puberty, childbirth, pregnancy, and breastfeeding. All of these events will change the levels of hormones within a woman's body. We won't focus on irregular cycles during puberty as that is an age where the body is always going through changes and the hormones in a woman's body can take a couple of years to regulate themselves.

What do your contraceptives with hormones do to your body? Your hormonal birth control can also impact your menstrual cycle. For example, intrauterine devices (IUDs) are the most common method of birth control that can cause a woman to experience heavy cramping and bleeding.

However, it is not always birth control or life changes that affect our menstrual cycles. Sometimes it is our unhealthy habits that mess with the hormones in our body. If you are not treating yourself in the right way, your body will take it out on you in many ways, and often that includes your menstrual cycle. Bad health habits don't always include the way that you eat and can vary. Take a look at some of these bad habits we might have or illnesses and disorders we experience that can and do affect the menstrual cycle:

- Emotional stress

- Extreme weight loss or gain

- Eating disorders that include bulimia and anorexia

- Marathon running (or other forms of extreme endurance exercising)

So, what can you do to lessen the impact your unhealthy lifestyle habits have on your fertility? You want to live and maintain a lifestyle that is healthy. I don't mean you have to give up marathon running if that is your thing, however, you need to start making healthier choices for you. This can be hard if you are experiencing a time of significant stress or find yourself battling with a disorder. Remember that there are always people to reach out to. They can be friends, family, or even healthcare professionals.

Make sure that you exercise regularly so that you can keep a healthy body mass index (BMI) and keep your stress levels down. Also, ensuring that you are eating right and maintaining a balanced diet will help you keep your hormones in check.

If the cause lies with your hormonal birth control, you should seek out the advice of your doctor. Similarly, if you struggle with a disorder such as anorexia, then you need to lean on healthcare professionals to help you find your path back to health again.

Polycystic Ovary Syndrome (PCOS) is another hormonal problem that leads to irregular menstrual cycles. PCOS can be linked to obesity, however, this is not always the case. If you suffer from PCOS then you will not ovulate, which renders you infertile. PCOS is a condition that results in small polyps or cysts on a woman's ovaries, and you should seek out the advice of a medical professional to help you combat this problem. PCOS is a very common problem, affecting over 5 million of the American woman population. A healthcare professional might recommend a form of hormonal therapy or the removal of the cysts in order to help regulate your cycles.

Being extremely overweight or obese can also affect your menstrual cycle. If you safely lose some of the weight, you might see a return to regular menstrual cycles and you might start ovulating again.

There are other health concerns that could cause issues with irregular menstrual cycles such as cancer of the cervix or uterus. These types of cancer will also cause unnatural and unusual bleeding during odd times of your cycle. Thyroid issues also affect a woman's cycles. Sometimes a healthcare professional might want to evaluate your thyroid gland to make sure you don't suffer from a thyroid disorder when it comes to your irregular cycles.

Endometriosis can also impact your monthly cycles. This condition leaves you with endometrial cells that grow outside and around the uterus. These cells should normally grow on the inside. While this cell growth is not an indication of cancer, it can lead to pain and irregular cycles for women. You could also suffer tissue damage if endometriosis is left unchecked.

Pelvic Inflammatory Disease (PID) is an easily treatable infection that occurs inside a woman's reproductive system. While it is a very common complication from STIs for women, it can be rather serious and should be looked at right away. When detected in time, antibiotics can be used to help treat PID. However, once it spreads, PID can destroy the uterus and fallopian tubes. Not only will this cause infertility, but it is also extremely painful and the pain can go on for a long time. If you find that you bleed between your periods or especially after sexual intercourse then you need to go to a doctor and get tested. You don't want a smaller problem to develop into a bigger problem due to lack of treatment.

I know that all of that seemed extremely scary to read about, however, it is important to understand the factors that contribute to irregular menstrual cycles and how to combat them. Without understanding, you will be left in the dark and an easily treatable problem can turn into a lifelong journey of pain and suffering from infertility. This is why tracking your ovulation is your best friend because it can help indicate to you the minute there is any problem with your reproductive system.

Strap into your seats ladies, because I am going to tackle another serious issue that not many women are aware of — anovulation. You already know that ovulation is when your ovaries release an egg or two eggs in the hopes of getting pregnant. Sometimes, while a woman might experience a regular cycle, her egg will not mature and therefore she will not ovulate since the egg never gets released from the ovaries. When this happens, it is referred to as anovulation. A woman who experiences anovulation will also experience irregular menstrual cycles or even the complete lack of a menstrual cycle or period.

Anovulation can cause serious issues when it comes to infertility. It can be caused by a series of different conditions or medications. These issues normally affect your hormone levels.

Anovulation can occur for merely a cycle or two and then the woman's body goes back to its regular cycle. However, there are times where it becomes a chronic issue and leads to infertility.

Anovulation can be very frustrating to deal with. If you suspect this is your problem as you begin to track your monthly cycle, I recommend purchasing the ovulation prediction kits. They can be found at most grocery stores or pharmacies and they can help you confirm your suspicions about your ovulation phase of the menstrual cycle.

Your most common culprit for anovulation is hormonal contraceptives. Remember though, that if avoiding pregnancy is your goal with hormonal contraceptives that they are doing their job by causing anovulation. Hormonal contraceptives will stop your hormones from producing mature eggs, and therefore, your ovaries will not have any eggs to release to begin your ovulation phase. Some types of birth control that are commonly known to cause these issues are:

- The Birth Control Patch — this is placed on any part of your body that you choose each week to prevent pregnancy.

- The Birth Control Pill — this is taken daily by mouth to prevent pregnancy.

- The Birth Control Implant — this is placed under the

skin of a woman's upper arm and prevents pregnancy for 3 years.

- The Vaginal Ring — this is placed inside the vagina and lasts for one month to prevent pregnancy.

- The Birth Control Shot — this is an arm injection that gets received once every 12 weeks to prevent a woman from getting pregnant.

- Intrauterine Device (IUD) — this can be hormonal or non-hormonal, for this chapter we are focusing on the hormonal IUD which is placed inside the uterus and prevents pregnancy for up to 5 years.

The above hormonal contraceptives will stop the ovaries' job of growing and releasing mature eggs for fertilization. I mentioned that there is a non-hormonal IUD which is commonly called the copper IUD. This device does not have hormones in it and therefore does not cause anovulation, it merely stops the sperm from being able to reach the mature egg.

It is not always birth control that interferes with a woman's ovulation. Ask your doctor about all side effects of prescribed medications as these can also affect your hormones. The negative side effects of other medications can impact your fertility. For example, drugs that are non-steroidal anti-inflammatory medications might seem harmless enough. These can come in the form of pain relievers like ibuprofen and can cause anovulation if you take them consistently, especially for a period longer than 10 days (Berry 2017).

Homeopathic and natural home remedies might sound amazing when you first hear about them and try them, however, there are herbs and plants that contain hormones that affect your own natural hormonal balance. Make sure that you are educated about any natural supplements or home remedies before taking them if you are trying to get pregnant. Alternatively, also consult your doctor to make sure it is okay to use.

You might be surprised by the usual everyday items you use that can cause anovulation. It can become quite frustrating to learn about all the ways that you are impacting your body but knowledge is true power. Without this knowledge, you wouldn't be able to take your own fertility health into your hands. Personally, I think learning about what makes your body tick is very important. Let's take a look at more common items you might be using that can cause anovulation.

Take a closer look at the skin creams and other prescribed and non-prescribed topical creams and liquids that you use. Some of these products have estrogen and progesterone in them. Particularly those anti-aging creams we all love so much. Estrogen and progesterone are helpful with many other issues such as wrinkles that women face and are even present in medications that are used to combat premenstrual syndrome (PMS). The topical products you use are absorbed through your skin and into your body where the additional hormones wreak havoc with your hormones that are already present. This, in turn, causes an imbalance which leads to anovulation.

Steroids are common prescription medications that are given out for various different ailments and cuts. Their main job is to reduce inflammation. Your steroids are also a hormone, and they will mess with your body and the balance of hormones nature has already set out for you. For example, a study was done and an article then published regarding women with Rheumatic disease. Half of the women who received a steroid shot for treatment later found that they had irregular menstrual cycles (Berry 2017).

Epilepsy and seizure medication are important lifesavers. However, they can do damage to a woman's reproductive system. Always consult a doctor regarding trying to get pregnant if you are on epilepsy medication. The reason for this is that not only does the medication interfere with your natural menstrual cycle, it can also cause birth deformities or disabilities in unborn babies (Berry 2017).

Cancer treatment is rough. Ask anyone who's been through it and they won't tell you it was a walk in the park. It can be even harder when you are a woman who has lost her fertility due to necessary life-saving treatment. The harsh radiation, chemotherapy, and other combination of cancer drugs can destroy a woman's ovaries. And by destroy, I mean irreversible damage. Unfortunately, there is little to do if this is the situation you encounter but there are plenty of options that you can discuss and should discuss with your doctor beforehand if you wish to have children in the future and are of childbearing age.

As with issues that cause irregular cycles, they overlap into anovulation problems. For example. PCOS that affects millions of women worldwide, thyroid issues, hypothalamus issues, and a host of other medical problems can cause both irregular cycles and anovulation. While they may seem like similar concepts, there are some key differences in how they affect the body and the reproductive system.

Anovulation really becomes a problem when a woman is trying to get pregnant, however, if there is no reason for you to miss your ovulation phase, you will want to consult your doctor about what other issues might be impacting your menstrual cycle.

As there are so many different outside influences and variables that contribute to a woman's anovulation there is no one cure-all solution. Unfortunately, it may take some trial and error or additional testing before the causative factor of anovulation is found. Luckily, because it is mostly a product of a hormone imbalance, anovulation is usually easily treatable.

Stress

I know it can be frustrating when you are trying to get pregnant and all around you is an onslaught of women who seem to get pregnant merely by breathing in the fresh spring air. Maybe you are at your wit's end and tired because you have done all the testing, the trying, the waiting, hormones, and a mass of other ideas in an attempt to get pregnant and it simply is not working. Around you are a plethora of well-meaning friends who simply want you to relax and take a step out of your stress zone because that's exactly what your baby fever has driven you to — stress.

As unsolicited and unwelcome as the advice may be for you to relax, sometimes there is great wisdom in those words. With the ever-revolving research being done around fertility and the recent breakthroughs the medical community has made when it comes to fertility, it is not surprising that new evidence has linked infertility issues to stress. There was a study published in 2010 that showed that women who experienced high levels of stress struggled with infertility (Johnson 2010). The reason for this is that when your body enters periods of extreme duress, an enzyme called alpha-amylase is produced, and this enzyme interferes with the reproductive process. In the study, the researchers gathered samples of their saliva over a period of six or more menstrual cycles to see their levels of the alpha-amylase enzymes. It was found that those who had higher levels of the enzyme suffered from a 12 percent reduction in the ability to get pregnant compared to women with lower levels of the enzyme. It is important to note that these women who underwent periods of stress had no prior infertility issues.

While more research is being conducted on the effects stress has on fertility, we all know that stress can negatively impact the body. There are physical ailments that are a product of stress that plague our bodies. So, is it really that difficult to believe that stress impacts our fertility?

While there are women who manage to get pregnant under intensely stressful situations, this is not the case for everyone. Often an obsession or concern over infertility causes stress that interferes with conception. This additional level of stress wreaks havoc on the body and leaves a woman struggling to conceive. There are other stress hormones such as cortisol that will impact the female reproductive system by causing anovulation. Stress management can mean the difference between fertility and infertility. If you think that you are over-stressed or over-extended, it is time to step back and reduce your levels of stress. Research that was published in 2003 indicated that women who went through therapy to reduce their levels of stress were able to start ovulating again (Johnson 2010). Stress really does hinder your reproductive function. There are some key things you can do to lessen the load on your plate. If you think stress is the main culprit in your life right now, try using the steps below to reduce that stress:

- Lean on your significant other. Men and women handle stress differently. For women, social support is one of the easiest ways to find stress relief. During times of infertility, women might become hyper-focused on the issue and cause strain between them and their partner. Ask for your partner's help during this time. Don't bring all the attention to the infertility issue but rather, focus on doing things together that form a better bond or that remind you why you two are together in the first place. Do this at least once a week. Limit the focus on the elephant in the room and bring it back to your partner. Ask for their help with this to keep you on track as well. If you do want to talk about fertility issues or pregnancy-related problems, limit the discussion to a set time limit you both agree on so that it does not consume the relationship.

- Change your attitude toward pregnancy. Don't go in with the misconception that everyone around you is getting pregnant and you are still struggling. This will add to your levels of distress, and you know it's not true. You know there are other women in this world battling their own wars with infertility. Keep reminding yourself that fertility specialists and guides like this exist for a reason because you are not the only woman going through these troubles.

- Get some exercise. Keep doing those things that you found enjoyment in before pregnancy consumed your world. Don't let getting pregnant become your entire being. You are still a person and an individual who took pleasure in many activities before. If you love long walks take them, if painting is your poison then pick up that paintbrush. When you take part in an activity you love doing, then you create an aura of happiness and boost serotonin in your brain. This can only be a good thing as you keep those stress hormones away.

- Sometimes writing it out helps. Get a journal and write about how you are feeling and what you are experiencing. If you want to keep the journal for memories go for it, alternatively, you can work on destroying the pages as a release of frustration.

- Meditate, focus on relaxing rather than stressing. This is a really easy one, which is what also makes it one of the hardest ones. Set at least two times a day where you can spend between 5 to 10 minutes focusing on nothing but your place of relaxation. This can be any location in your world where you feel completely at peace. For some people, this is a beach, for others this might be the forest, or even their very own living room. The idea is to focus on this area and let your body immerse itself as if it was present in that area. You will feel your heart rate decrease as you enter this state of relaxation, and this is what you want. Meditation can bring you back to yourself.

- Sometimes you need group support. Or even merely one on one counseling. Don't be afraid to seek out help and understanding from other people around you. You might find great community and resources from people who can take an objective stance and help you work through your feelings of confusion, frustration, and sadness. If you don't know where to begin looking for support, reach out to "resolve.org". This is an affiliate of the National Infertility Association and will have an avenue of support for you.

Brief Recap

I know this chapter might have seemed scary. It contained a lot of issues that relate to infertility and a lot of things you might be doing to indirectly influence your bad health. I want you to take a moment and remember that the purpose of this chapter was not to scare you but to educate and motivate you. I want it to serve as a light at the end of the tunnel, letting you know that: Yes! There are things you can do to improve your health and your chances of conception. As you go into the next few chapters which will help guide you into those healthy lifestyle choices, keep in mind some of the things you might be able to change now.

- Stress impacts your fertility by creating high levels of enzymes and hormones that impact your ovulation phase.

- Everyday medications, topical creams, and even steroids can have hormones in them that change the way your reproductive system functions. Always consult a doctor before you start a new medication if you are trying to get pregnant.

- Bad fertility health can be caused by both things you are doing actively or inactively. Education is the key to making bad health become good health. You can't fix a problem if you don't know what it is.

- Other issues like PCOS and endometriosis can cause

major fertility issues for women. Sometimes a hormonal treatment works, other times surgery might be needed to correct the problem.

- Anovulation is the absence of a mature egg being released during the time you should be ovulating. Sometimes, it happens for only a cycle or two, and other times, it can last indefinitely.

- Irregular menstrual cycles are more common than many people think. Normally, they are considered irregular if they surpass a period of longer than 35 days.

Chapter 5: Why Good Health Is Extremely Important for Fertility

In the previous section, we covered exactly why you want to practice good health habits. When you partake in unhealthy habits, you can create problems with your reproductive organs and their systems for managing your fertility. This isn't the end of the world though as you can turn things around and begin practicing good health immediately!

Good health is important for your fertility because it helps ensure that your reproductive processes are functioning as they should. This means that you give your body one less thing to worry about or manage when it comes to your fertility. Take a look at the benefits of living a healthy lifestyle and what your future lifestyle should include as you continue on the path of reproductive improvement.

Benefits of Living Healthy

Taking care of your reproductive system is incredibly important, especially in the context of fertility. You want your hormones to be balanced so that your ovulation phase occurs as it should. You want to feel happy and content and like you have the energy to conquer the world every day. This is what living a healthy lifestyle can provide for you.

A healthy lifestyle includes more than exercise and nutrition, even though those two aspects are an important part of living healthy. However, don't let your mental health escape you as this is also a vital part of living healthy and maintaining a healthy lifestyle. If you suffer from depression or other mental health issues then it is best to work with your doctor to help bring you back to a place where you are maintaining your mental health.

You will need to make "sacrifices" as you move towards a healthier lifestyle such as quitting alcohol drinking and tobacco use. The benefits that come to you with a healthier lifestyle are immeasurable, truly.

Let's take a look at one of the best aspects of living a healthy life — an improved mood. This has a huge impact on where you are mentally. It has been proven that exercise helps produce endorphins — the chemical in the brain that leaves you feeling refreshed and happy. Both diet and exercise are tied to a release of endorphins. They improve your outlook not only on your internal health but also on your external appearance. Your mood will be boosted because you are experiencing less self-doubt and more self-esteem.

Your improved mood also requires more than diet and exercise. Keeping up with your social connections and making new ones can help release happy chemicals through your body. Humans are social creatures and social stimulation is part of living a healthy lifestyle. Staying connected and socializing can be as simple as calling a friend or volunteering for your favorite cause.

A healthy lifestyle also prevents diseases and other serious conditions. Often times these conditions can have a direct effect on fertility or your ability to carry a baby to term. By living a healthy lifestyle, you can avoid preventable problems like strokes, heart disease, and high cholesterol and blood pressure. Staying fit and active can help you fight against depression, diabetes, arthritis, metabolic syndrome, and other diseases that affect your fertility.

Future Lifestyle Habits

When you follow healthy lifestyle habits then your overall health is improved. This is beneficial since your health is linked to your fertility, in both you and any potential partner of yours. It can be difficult to eliminate those unhealthy habits and replace them with healthier ones, but it should be one of your first steps as you take an active leap toward parenthood. You might struggle with making these changes and adaptations in your life, but I am here to help guide you onto the right road. When you are focusing on making a healthy lifestyle for you and your partner, keep the following tips in mind and start to change your life to adopt these healthier habits. Not only will your bodies thank you, but your potential future children will as well. Remember that even if you are going through hormonal treatments for fertility or IVF programs, good health can also mean the difference between success and failure.

1. Before you do anything else you need to make sure that you are giving your body the right nutrition and the nutrients that it needs. A healthy diet means that your body is receiving a well-balanced proportion of fruits, vegetables, and proteins. Pregnancy requires a lot of nutrients and a pregnancy ready body is no different. By eating healthy, you also ensure that you maintain the ideal weight and shape for your potential pregnancy. It might be hard if you have certain dietary restrictions, however, there are ways to still get your nutrients and maintain a balanced diet despite these restrictions. Talk

to your doctor to help come up with the right meal assortment that works for you and your body. It is helpful if both you and your partner participate in the same dietary choices.

2. This might be a touchy subject, but it is one that does need to be explored. You need to control your weight when you plan on getting pregnant (it is helpful to always make sure that you have a healthy BMI). Being both underweight and overweight has its own set of problems that it brings to the fertility field. When you have a healthy BMI, then your ovulation phase is more likely to occur as it should and your risk for anovulation due to weight concerns is extremely low. As unfortunate as the statistics are to report, women who are considered extremely overweight or obese are far more likely to experience the devastating effects of a miscarriage than those women who have healthy BMIs. Maintaining weight might be hard and can require a support system. You can find support in a partner, a family, or even a health professional like a nutritionist who is there to make sure you are at your healthiest. While this might sound discouraging, if you are overweight, I want you to keep in mind that a small weight loss in the margins of 5 to 10 percent of your current body weight will vastly improve fertility issues.

3. Folic acid and iodine supplements will be your best friend. This is especially true if you are going through any hormonal fertility treatments to improve your fertility. Normally, you will also take these supplements during your first trimester of pregnancy. You can easily get these in most pharmacies but make sure that you stick to the recommended dosage.

4. Keep your body in shape by exercising. Create a plan for regular exercise. Don't push or overexert yourself as this can have negative effects, but moderate exercise for 30 minutes a day can help improve your body and release positive endorphins into your body. This also helps reduce those feelings of stress in your body. There is a balance to exercise. If you are in peak physical shape and an avid exerciser, consider lessening the amount you exercise slightly so that you don't overexert yourself.

5. Cut out smoking and avoid people/places where you will be exposed to secondary smoke. If you smoke then you will surely have a harder time conceiving. Studies have shown that smoking drastically impacts ovulation and the ability to release a mature egg for fertilization during ovulation. This goes for both male and female partners, as smoking has been proven to lower male sperm counts and impact the success of fertility treatments such as IVF. When you smoke as a woman, you can affect your body in such negative ways that early menopause might be prompted, your ovaries will age and suffer damage, and the chances of miscarriage also increase. As you smoke, keep in mind that your risk of cervical cancer increases and any damage to your cervix or fallopian tubes will render you unable to carry the fertilized egg to term. Quitting smoking is the best thing you can do for your body.

6. Double-check all medications that you are on or are taking with your doctor. Remember that certain medications can impact your hormonal balance and shift your reproductive processes on their head. Discuss all medications you plan on taking — yes, even over the counter medications — to ensure that you are still giving yourself the best chance at conception.

7. Stop drinking alcohol excessively or frequently. I am not talking about your one glass of red wine with dinner here and there but rather mass and unhealthy drinking. Excessive drinking can not only cause miscarriage and fertility problems but birth defects if you are able to successively conceive. Alcohol can be the cause of anovulation and irregular menstrual cycles. If you are planning on getting pregnant or undergoing any fertility treatments, both you and your partner should monitor your alcohol intake and change habits as necessary. If you are trying to conceive, I recommend that you cut out all alcohol completely to heighten your chances.

8. Slow down your caffeine consumption. When you consume excess amounts of caffeine (this includes coffee, tea, and other products), you are adding stress onto your adrenals. Your blood sugar also takes a wild trip and doesn't settle down for a few hours. Excessive consumption of caffeine can prolong the amount of time it takes a woman to conceive. Try limiting yourself or even entirely cutting out all coffee and caffeinated drinks when you are trying to conceive.

9. I know this one goes without saying, but for the sake of your future health and to make sure all the bases are covered I am going to mention that you should stop or avoid all recreational drugs. The reason for this is because they do have a direct effect on fertility, and drugs like cocaine and even marijuana (not that the world likes to discuss this) can impact the reproductive systems of both males and females. Do yourself a favor and avoid them altogether when you are trying to get pregnant.

10. I just completed an entire section on stress reduction, so I won't belabor my points here. However, for the success of a future healthy lifestyle, make sure that you are partaking in activities that reduce your stress and allow you to live a happier and lighter life. Infertility can be very stressful, so head back up to chapter four if you need some more resources on how to handle the stress you have and turn it into a more positive feeling. Remember, you are a person and you should dedicate time away from fertility talk and focus on you and your enjoyment too.

The main point of this list is to help you and your partner get your body ready for a baby! You can do this by setting your mind to it and being determined about your health. Throw out those reminders of your past lifestyle and prepare yourself for a healthier future. You can do this, you merely need to remain dedicated!

Brief Recap

Is there any shortage to the list of benefits that come from living a healthy lifestyle? Are there any genuine reasons other than self-indulgence to avoid living a healthy life? Not really. Your most important job is to care for your body and the future baby that you hope to conceive. Even if your main goal is not to conceive but to understand your body better, your health should still be your first goal.

- Keep in mind that eating and exercising right is essential to maintaining both internal and external health.

- When you keep a healthy lifestyle, you fight off other diseases that could impact your fertility. You take the stress off your reproductive system when you maintain a healthy hormone balance and an improved mood.

- Boosted energy and mood are directly associated with feeling good about yourself and feeling healthy. When you exercise right, you release endorphins that assist in an improved mood.

- There are many habits you can start cutting out right now to prepare yourself for a healthier future. Stop smoking, cut out caffeine, and limit your alcohol intake. These are the first and most important steps you can take.

- Clean out your cupboards and pantry of all unhealthy food and stock yourself up with nutritious food that is going to serve your body well. Removing the temptation to eat unhealthily is half the battle.

Chapter 6: Dieting Do's and Don'ts

It's all well and good to tell you to eat a healthy diet, but what does that diet look like? Sometimes the food that is healthy to eat is not the best food to promote fertility. Marketing can also come across as deceptive, and while we may think that we are eating a delicious and well-balanced meal, we are really missing out on the real nutrition that we need.

When we talk about food items that are safe and unsafe, it can start to become a little complicated. I want to provide you some clarity and also make it easy for you to identify what you should incorporate into your diet and what you should do your best to avoid or exclude from your diet. It might still be hard for you to believe that your diet has a huge impact on your fertility but hold on to your seats because I am about to change your perception about the way that you eat!

How Your Diet Affects Fertility

I am sure that you have heard the telltale signs of pregnancy where women avoid certain types of foods they believe are unhealthy for a growing baby. This commonly occurs after a woman gets pregnant. However, we often skip over the part about a woman's diet before she gets pregnant. Making key diet changes before pregnancy is incredibly important. Your diet plays a massive role in your fertility and should not be overlooked.

When we talk about diet and fertility, the main area of focus is going to be the way that your diet interferes with ovulation.

You need your hormones to be balanced out and functioning at an optimal level in order for ovulation to occur as it should every cycle. However, having a poorly structured diet can mess with this hormonal balance and therefore disrupt your period of ovulation. So, the best way to ensure that your diet is not the deciding factor on if you can or cannot get pregnant is to correct it while trying to conceive. You can reduce your risk of suffering infertility by making a few smart dietary changes.

I know you have heard your fill from me about your estrogen and progesterone hormones. I get it. You understand their importance in your cycle. However, when it comes to infertility based on dietary concerns, the other important hormone I am going to be discussing is insulin. When you have an excess amount of the insulin hormone in your body, you risk anovulation. Not only do you risk your eggs not maturing and releasing, but you also have an increased risk for cysts to form on your ovaries. When your diet consists of high levels of carbohydrates, complex sugars, and lots of starch then you are at risk of having too high levels of insulin. The reason for this is that overeating white breads and flours or even potatoes and rice prompts the pancreas to begin producing more insulin so that the carbohydrates being consumed can be metabolized.

If your ultimate goal is to help your body ovulate correctly with each cycle and increase your fertility then your first step should be to limit your consumption of carbohydrates and sugars. You want to maintain the appropriate insulin levels, and so eliminating trans fats as well as french fries and margarines can help you as well. I will go more in-depth about specific foods at one moment, but you should pay special attention to what you are consuming. Avoid foods that say half-fat or seem processed. Natural foods are always best for you. They are best for your body as well. It might seem like a good idea to eat that low carb butter now, but in the long run, it might mess with your reproductive system.

A surprising dietary change that you might not be prepared for is to eliminate most fruits from your diet. Of course, it is a healthier alternative to that chocolate cake you want to put in your grocery cart and a far safer option if your sweet tooth is bothering you. However, fruits are high in sugars and can create excess insulin as well. Practice moderation when you eat them.

The best thing you can do for yourself is to remove those fancy sports drinks and other sugary drinks like sodas. Place a greater emphasis on drinking water and non-caffeinated herbal teas instead, this will help maintain your body's insulin balance.

The concern with your diet and fertility is not all about the excess of the insulin hormone. Your body needs vital vitamins and nutrients that it gets from the foods you consume daily. Most marketed and pre-packaged foods lack these necessary vitamins. When you suffer from a deficiency in vitamin D, iron, iodine, and selenium, the first place you should look at is your diet. These are necessary for ovulation to occur and lacking them will prevent your ovulation from occurring. Some women take a multivitamin to help increase these levels when they are trying to get pregnant, but you can also naturally control this through your diet by making smart choices about the foods you consume. Having a healthy diet should be at the top of your priority list.

Diets That Promote Fertility

Okay, so, now you know how important your diet is to ovulation, what next? Hormones are finicky things, aren't they? There are certain foods you can eat or increase your intake of that are good for your body and help promote fertility. This means that they help your body get ready for ovulation.

Quinoa is a great grain that you can consume in preparation for pregnancy. It is gluten-free and one of the staple foods you should introduce into your diet when trying to help your fertility health. Many people are not aware that quinoa can help actively control their blood sugar levels. Your body takes longer to digest quinoa since it has such a high fiber content as well as a higher protein content. You can also use brown rice or whole grain breads as they tend to have high fiber content too. By helping your blood sugar levels remain in check, quinoa helps eliminate the risk of the pesky overproduction of insulin in your body.

If you love fish then wild salmon is your perfect source of omega-3. Omega-3 is a healthy fat, and it is a basic building block of those necessary hormones you need for ovulation. The other thing that wild salmon benefits is your brain function which will help you feel better each day. The healthy fats from omega-3 can also help you if you suffer from painful menstrual cycles. Not everyone loves fish though, or you may be a vegetarian, the good news is that walnuts and flax seeds are excellent sources of Omega-3.

Dark and leafy greens like spinach can provide you with your iron and folate. Iron is essential to your menstrual cycle, especially during your active bleeding phase. Not only does it help you during menstruation, but it also acts as a support to ovulation and ensuring those eggs mature well. Anemia can be a real concern as you get pregnant or want to get pregnant, so focusing on increasing your iron intake can prevent you from developing anemia. Folate is an important nutrient, particularly during the first trimester of your pregnancy. The reason is that it will help your baby with its brain and neural development. It also supports heart development, and since your baby's heart starts beating at four weeks, you can see where it is incredibly important to make sure your baby has the necessary nutrients available to it immediately after conception.

Ignore all of those fat-free and low-fat marketing schemes and invest in some whole fat dairy products. Greek yogurt is a great source of nutrients, but it has to be whole fat. Whole fat dairy products have many necessary nutrients that we require, even for ourselves alone. Full-fat Greek yogurt can provide you the protein, vitamin D, and calcium you need. Vitamin D plays a crucial part in making sure that your sexual hormones are balanced and your menstrual cycles are regular. Organic is always best as you avoid any added additives or hormones — as I have already covered, you do not need to add additional hormones to your body unless this is a treatment from your doctor.

While fruits are not necessary, they can be a hard thing to give up for those with a sweet tooth. And if you are anything like me, you feel less guilty snacking on a strawberry than you do a bar of chocolate. Fruits that are bright in color like blueberries, pomegranates, strawberries, and raspberries contain vitamin C, fiber, and folate. However, their main benefit is the antioxidants that they are chock full of. These antioxidants are known to boost fertility since they repair and reduce damage to reproductive cells.

Ignore the association of the oyster with an aphrodisiac for one moment. Oysters are considered a superfood when it comes to fertility. While you should not eat raw oysters during your pregnancy, before pregnancy you should consume them for the high amounts of zinc that they can provide to you. I am not an oyster fan, so I was thankful to find that pumpkin seeds can provide a similar level of zinc as oysters. Zinc is important to fertility as it helps boosts the reproductive system.

Iron, fiber, and folate will never stop being important during and before pregnancy. You can find these in lentils. Not only do they give you a great source of protein but they provide necessary nutrients for a pre-pregnancy body. You might be wondering why fiber is so important to the fertility process, doesn't it only help your digestive system? Interestingly enough, fiber also gets rid of those extra hormones your body doesn't need.

I highly suggest that you go to your nearest grocery store, buy away, and bon appetit!

Diets That Hinder Fertility

Now that you know what you can eat for fertility, it can be harder to determine what to avoid. There are so many foods out there that do hinder fertility. I don't want you to find that you are eating something you think is good for you but is harming you in the long run. While it is critical that you make dietary changes when you are pregnant, making them before you are pregnant can help you adjust a lot faster and benefit your reproductive system if you are trying to conceive.

While a big part of eating right is eating the correct foods, your more important job is understanding what is bad for you and your potential baby. You want to avoid those artificial foods stuffed with fake hormones and synthetic ingredients. If you find that packaged and processed foods are a large part of your diet right now, don't freak out. It's okay. Remember change can be made at any point and you will find benefits from it. Now that you are armed with the knowledge you need, you can correct the choices you were making before.

The number one item that you need to avoid when pregnant is fish with high mercury content. Here's the thing about mercury — it is detrimental to your nervous system. When you eat it often before pregnancy, your body will store the mercury up and this can negatively affect your baby when you do manage to conceive. If you know you want to have a baby in the next year or less then put away the fish with high mercury content (mostly tuna and swordfish) and find a good replacement like wild salmon.

Trans fats are easily found in your favorite chips and those instant microwaveable popcorn pouches the world loves so much. Fried foods are also a mecca for trans fats. These fats are bad because they promote inflammation in your body and create a resistance to insulin. You already know this is bad because excess insulin interferes with ovulation. In the worst-case scenario, the trans fats you consume will destroy your blood vessels. You might not think this is a major issue until you realize that your blood vessels are what carry the nutrients you need to your reproductive system.

Throw away all of the soda. Diet soda and regular soda. They lower fertility by increasing your risk of inflammation and creating critical metabolic changes in your body. The sodas that you consume also come in receptacles that contain chemicals that the carbonation eats away at and absorbs. Do yourself a favor and avoid them for you and your baby's health.

Any food that is high in sugar content and will make your blood sugar rise quickly should be avoided. Especially when they are not paired with foods like quinoa which will stop this spike. You don't want a spike in blood sugar to change your hormonal balance and cause anovulation. This means to avoid a majority of carbohydrates, particularly refined ones.

Avoid drinking alcohol. Before, during, and after pregnancy. Sometimes it is hard to consider cutting out all alcohol from your diet. If this is where you stand and you enjoy that glass of red wine too much, do not drink more than seven drinks per week. That is one drink a day. The reason for this is that your alcohol habit will take away the vitamin B in your body which is necessary for fertility.

All low-fat dairy should be avoided at all costs. These products have androgens which are male hormones. It could prompt your body to continue to produce more androgens, and then your menstrual cycle could be disrupted entirely.

Avoid processed meats like deli meat. This includes smoked fish. The reason is that they are very likely to come into contact with listeria. If you cannot avoid processed meat, at least heat it up so that you give yourself a chance of killing the bacteria that might live on the meat.

All unpasteurized cheeses like gorgonzola, camembert, and brie will also be prone to listeria contamination. Avoid them completely. There is also a link between unpasteurized cheeses and miscarriage. When in doubt? Avoid.

My sushi lovers out there will not be happy when I say that, if you are trying to conceive, you should avoid all raw meat, raw eggs, and raw seafood. These raw animal products can contain so many different bacteria and contaminants that will not only infect any potential fetus but also negatively affect your reproductive system. This includes those delicious carpaccios that you like. Skip the raw products and get a nice well-cooked chicken breast instead.

Brief Recap

There are so many do's and don'ts when it comes to healthy eating and healthy living. Sometimes it can be hard to keep track of what food lies on which list. The biggest thing to remember is that your body really is your temple in the period before conception. What you put into your body to nourish it can mean the difference between fertility and infertility.

- Make sure that all dairy products you consume are full-fat. Organic full-fat Greek yogurt is a great choice before and during pregnancy. Avoid unpasteurized soft cheeses.

- Make sure that you don't eat any raw animal products and veer on the side of caution when it comes to deli meats. Always cook your food so that you can ensure any potentially harmful bacteria have had a chance to die off.

- Insulin is a hormone in your body that can prompt anovulation to occur if there is an excess in your body. An excess of insulin is normally prompted when you eat foods that are high in sugars.

- Quinoa and any other brown rice or brown bread will help give your body the necessary fiber it needs to fight off potential blood sugar spikes you might experience.

- Fruits are not the best thing for you because they do have high sugar content, but colorful fruits like blueberries are high in antioxidants that benefit the reproductive system.

- Fish like tuna and swordfish are high in mercury and should be avoided at all costs. They can negatively affect the neural development of a fetus.

Chapter 7: Natural Birth Control

Did you know that there are methods of natural birth control? This means that you don't always have to rely on hormones to prevent pregnancy. This guide is not meant only for women who wish to conceive but also for those who wish to control their own health and not be subservient to the hormones that wreak havoc on our bodies.

If you are a woman between the ages of 16 and 45, the odds are that you have at some point in your life experienced hormonal birth control. If you are one of the lucky few who have not, or one of the lucky few who have had no adverse side effects, then kudos. However, we always have more that we can learn about ourselves, the medical world that tells us what to do, and how to balance all this information.

Negative Impact of Hormonal Birth Control

It is no secret that the hormonal birth control pill that you take has some severe negative impacts on your body. Most hormonal contraceptives contain estrogen and progesterone which is released in your body when you consume them or place them in your body. When your body has super high levels of either hormone, it will prevent your ovaries from releasing an egg. When this happens, it prevents you from getting pregnant.

The other job that higher levels of progesterone do is to mess with your cervical fluid. It makes your cervical fluid thicker than usual so that the sperm struggle to make it into the uterus.

There are several different types of birth control which I covered earlier in this guide, and each one has various side effects that can negatively impact your body. For example, if you use the IUD Mirena then there is a chance that your menstruation will be shorter than usual. Some women take birth control to lessen the effects that their menstrual cycles can have on their bodies as sometimes the side effects lessen menstrual cramping. However, most hormonal birth control methods share certain symptoms that negatively affect different areas of our body.

It can take months or even years after you stop hormonal birth control for your body and its systems to go back to how they should normally function.

The most common side effects that affect your reproduction and sexual activity when you take hormonal birth control are:

- Breast tenderness

- Breast enlargement

- Vaginal irritation or inflammation

- Bleeding between menstruation

- Loss of menstruation

- An increased frequency of menstruation

- A decreased libido

There are times where heavy menstruation can occur for a period of longer than 7 days. If this happens, always stop your birth control and consult your doctor about this adverse side effect.

So, how exactly does hormonal birth control affect the different body systems? Let us start with your central nervous system and cardiovascular system. There are risks that, if you start taking hormonal contraceptives, your blood pressure can increase significantly and you could also risk blood clots. There are certain factors that raise the chances of you developing these issues while on birth control such as if you:

- Are a smoker

- Are over the age of 35

- Already have a heart condition or disease

- Already suffer from high blood pressure

- Have diabetes

The side effects that you experience from hormonal birth control are rather serious, and should they persist, you need to see a doctor about your concerns. In rare cases, you might experience severe pain in your head, weakness or numbness in your limbs, and trouble speaking. This indicates you might be suffering from a stroke. Seek medical help immediately. Always disclose your birth control as a medication that you are taking so that your doctors can prescribe your medication with that in mind.

Women who suffer from migraines can find that increased levels of estrogen rile migraines up and make them worse and more frequent. Changes in mood and depressive episodes are also not uncommon when taking hormonal methods of birth control. This is because the addition of new hormones into a balanced system causes chaos and affects more than your reproductive system.

Your digestive system is not safe from the harmful effects of birth control either. You may find that, shortly after taking birth control, your entire appetite changes. You might feel that you are eating more food, and you will see that you are gaining weight. There is evidence out there that links unexpected weight gain to birth control. Why is your eating pattern changing when birth control is introduced?

This is because your hormones help regulate almost everything that your body does, including its desire for food. When you introduce new hormones, there's a chance that you can affect the foods that you crave and the way that you eat. If you need or are adamant to remain on hormonal birth control, make sure that you are maintaining a healthy lifestyle and not making drastic unhealthy dietary changes.

You might experience additional feelings of being bloated or nauseated as you begin a hormonal contraceptive as well. Sometimes these feelings ease as your body gets adjusted to the birth control, other times they remain with you and you have to change your method of contraception.

Anyone with a history of gallstones should consult their doctor before taking birth control, as hormonal birth control can help these stones form faster and more frequently.

Your integumentary system is also affected by birth control. While one of the things that birth control advertises is control of and reductions in acne, there are women who find that their breakouts of acne worsen significantly while on birth control. There are rare cases of brown spotting happening over the skin after taking birth control.

It can be difficult and close to impossible for your doctor to predict how birth control will affect you and your body, which is why they might have you try out several different types of birth control before you settle on one that has side effects you can handle or don't yet notice.

You might find that abnormal and unusual hair growth occurs as a result of the hormones in your birth control. Your best bet is to discuss all of your options for birth control with a healthcare professional. Don't be shy about bringing up your concerns as well. Hormonal birth control is not necessary to prevent pregnancy, and if you don't have to negatively mess with your body, why do it?

Shortcuts to Charting

I know that I might have made charting seem like a lot of work and a lot of data to collect earlier on. When you get used to charting, this doesn't seem like so much information, but it can be overwhelming to someone who is newly entering the world of charts and menstrual cycles. Often people see the things they have to pay attention to when charting and they decide that charting is not for them.

Because I want to set you up for success with the FAM method, I want to introduce you to a little thing I like to call: Shortcut Charting.

Please remember that in your first month of charting, it is immeasurably important to get down all of the information regarding your BBT, cervical fluid, and cervical position. This is so that it builds up your habit of collecting the information. Also, the more information you miss, the less accurate your charts will be and you might be confused about your ovulation phase. I highly encourage you to fully chart your first month because it builds up your strength in charting and it helps you create good habits regarding checking your body.

Here's the thing. Once you get used to your body (this normally takes a few cycles) and you are aware of what to look out for, you can be less in-depth with your charting methods after you are sure you are in your ovulation phase.

While I do recommend a full year of cycle charting before delving into the shortcut method, what you do and how you do your charting is entirely up to you. When you first start charting, if you find that you are overwhelmed with all the information you need to record then you can try recording your data using different methods.

For example, when it comes to charting your basal body temperature. You do not have to do this during the week that you are actively menstruating. Your body's BBT will be unreliable during this time of your cycle anyway. The only time I suggest taking your temperature during the menstrual phase of your cycle is if your cycles are shorter than average and you have a risk of ovulating earlier. Those recordings will then be vital to help you decipher when you are and are not ovulating.

Also, once you know you are ovulating, you can ease up on taking your temperature. However, your previous readings need to be accurate and show a significant shift towards ovulation before you relax on taking your temperature. If you are unsure then I suggest you continue to record your temperature as it hardly takes time out of your day.

You also do not have to continue evaluating your cervical fluid once you know you are ovulating. Keep checking your cervical fluid until you make sure that you have one hundred percent confirmed ovulation — confirming it means you have recorded the correct temperature increase steadily and made sure that your other bodily signs point towards ovulation. Cervical fluid is something that you should be checking throughout your day, however, it is a very easy thing to check. Often you are already subconsciously noting the change in the consistency of this vaginal secretion. From the first day of your period until you confirm ovulation, you should still chart your cervical fluid.

Shortcut charting is not for everyone. There are some people who prefer to chart everything for the month, and there are some people who need to chart the entire month for other reasons. For example, if you are using the charting method to keep track of your health then it is important that you do record your fertility signs every single day. This is because a change in your cervical fluid can indicate an underlying health issue and you might miss that if you shortcut chart.

If you do not feel confident in your charting ability, then please, stick to charting all of your fertility signs until you do build that confidence. You need to know your body and be confident about what it is telling you before you try to shortcut chart.

Any illness can affect your signs, and therefore, this is a time where you should chart fully and accurately so that you can see the whole picture of what is going on for you. If you are unsure how your illness has affected your signs, make sure that you use protection during this cycle if you are avoiding pregnancy.

If you are only keeping track of one fertility sign, please do not shortcut chart. In order to shortcut chart, you need to be focusing on two different signs of fertility to make sure your readings and perceptions are accurate. It takes two fertility signs at the minimum to confirm ovulation.

Methods of Natural Birth Control

Did you know that you do not have to pump your body with hormones to achieve birth control methods? There are plenty of non-hormonal methods that you can use for birth control. For example, one of the more popular methods is known as the rhythm method. The rhythm method uses the ovulation cycle. Essentially, on the days that you are most fertile/ovulating, you abstain from any sexual intercourse.

However, there are a plethora of other natural birth control methods such as breastfeeding. For women that have given birth in the last 6 months and are exclusively breastfeeding — this means no solid foods or formula — the chance of getting pregnant is only 1 in 50 women. You must also make sure that you have not had a period since you gave birth as having a period may indicate that you have begun ovulating as well. You might have heard it called lactational infertility in the medical world, but many women do benefit from breastfeeding as a natural birth control method.

Withdrawal or the pull out method is another way to practice natural birth control. About 22 out of every 100 women get pregnant using the pull-out method as their main source of birth control. Withdrawal is where the penis is pulled out from the vagina before ejaculation occurs.

There is another natural method where you record your basal body temperature every day. Your temperature will drop just before your ovaries release your egg which indicates you have entered your fertility phase. Women who naturally control their fertility through their basal body temperature will abstain from sex while they know they are ovulating.

You might be surprised to learn that there are more options for natural birth control than the few mentioned above. There are natural health advocates who have a list of herbs that are supposedly effective at pregnancy prevention. Because natural methods and natural herbs and plants are preferable to synthetic chemicals, many people opt to try these out.

Please keep in mind when trying out these natural birth control methods listed below that they have not been approved as a method of birth control by any formal U.S. Food and Drug Administration. I recommend discussing options with your doctor before trying out one of the below methods to make sure that it is the right choice for you.

You might also want to try a lambskin condom. These are condoms that are natural and have not been treated with chemicals like the condoms you might find at your local grocery store.

Herbs you can try using are:

- Thistle: The Quinault and other Native Americans would historically drink a hot tea that was made with thistle in order to induce anovulation and prevent pregnancy.

- Stoneseed root: The Dakotas and the Shoshone were two Native American groups that made a cold mixture and drank it and then immediately inhaled the smoke from burning stoneseed root in order to create permanent sterility. Keep in mind this means that they would never get pregnant again.

- Wild carrot seed: There are women in parts of India who will eat one teaspoon of wild carrot seed after they have had sex. However, this method requires that one teaspoon is eaten right after sex, and again one teaspoon every day for the next 7 days so that implantation and conception do not occur. Some people suggest it as an abortive option as well for early unwanted pregnancies.

- Ginger root: There are natural health advocates who say that if you drink roughly 4 cups of ginger root tea every day for a period of exactly five days, you can start your menstrual phase. An alternative if you are missing fresh ginger root is to mix powdered ginger (roughly one teaspoon) into a cup of boiling water and drink it while it is still hot.

Brief Recap

Natural birth control methods gain popularity every day as women across the globe get tired of the negative side effects that hormonal birth control leaves them with. This chapter covered two major ideas. A shortcut to charting your cycle, and the idea of natural birth control that does not include charting. Let's take a closer look at some of the bigger ideas from this section.

- Hormonal birth control can cause high blood pressure and clots. In severe and rare cases, some women have suffered strokes due to birth control. Hormonal birth control aggravates migraines and other pre-existing medical issues because it increases the amount of hormones in your body.

- Shortcut charting works when you have an understanding of your body and what fertility looks like for you. You don't have to chart all of your signs every day, but you do have to make sure your charting is immaculate before you enter the phase of ovulation.

- There are methods such as withdrawal and the rhythm method that are used for natural birth control. They don't include the use of hormones.

- Lambskin condoms exist as a natural barrier against sperm reaching a mature egg in the uterus and have not been chemically treated like the condoms you buy in the grocery store.

- There are natural herbal remedies like thistle and stoneseed root that are used to cause infertility in women who do not want to get pregnant. Always consult your healthcare provider before proceeding with one of these methods.

Chapter 8: The Truth About Miscarriages

Miscarriage is hard to go through. This is true of both the mental and physical aspects of experiencing one. When most women first go through a miscarriage, they blame themselves and ask the question "why?" a lot.

If you have ever or are currently experiencing what a miscarriage is like, you will go through emotions such as anger, fear, guilt, and even depression. As women, we are told that our bodies serve one main purpose — to bear children. And the inability to do that often brings us great grief. I do want you to take a moment and remember that your life is important and that your life does not depend on the status of your reproductive system. Understanding more about miscarriage often helps women work through it.

Possible Reasons for Miscarriage

Miscarriage can happen for many different reasons. Some of the reasons are preventable with knowledge and other reasons are out of your scope of control. For example:

1. Chromosomal abnormalities are one of the most common reasons for miscarriages. This simply means that there was a problem during the formation of the embryo with either the chromosomes of the sperm or the mature egg. Sometimes chromosomal abnormalities can still result in conception and successful pregnancy,

other abnormalities are not viable for life. While these types of miscarriages can happen to any woman, they are more common in women over the age of 35. The reason for this is that as a woman ages, so do her eggs, and the possibility of them developing abnormalities increases as their age increases. A woman who is under the age of 20 has a 12 to 15 percent chance of experiencing a miscarriage. Unfortunately, those numbers nearly double the closer a woman gets to 40. Bear in mind that a miscarriage that occurs due to chromosomal abnormality had no chance of being saved. There is nothing that can prevent a situation like this one.

2. Diabetes is another common reason for miscarriage. Luckily for women who suffer from diabetes, there are methods to control what happens regarding your pregnancy. You must follow the strict advice of your doctor in this situation. The reason you need to closely listen to your doctor is that you need to ensure that your sugar is controlled at optimal levels while you are pregnant. If your diabetes is uncontrolled then you risk the chance of a miscarriage and even possible birth defects if you are able to carry to term. I suggest consulting with your doctor before getting pregnant so that you can come up with the best plan for your health before conceiving. You want your diabetes to be in a situation where it is well-controlled and where you can continue to monitor it and control it easily during the pregnancy.

3. Thyroid disorders can come in either hypo- or hyper-thyroidism. Hypo means low and hyper means high. The reason they are a disorder you want to watch in terms of

pregnancy is that these disorders can also lead to miscarriages. When you experience one of these disorders, it overproduces your hormones and puts stress on your body. Ovulation is therefore either suppressed or implantation becomes extremely difficult. You can even experience abnormal bleeding during a flare-up of your thyroid.

4. Your lifestyle habits are one of the biggest things you can control that often lead to miscarriages. This includes the use of alcohol while pregnant, smoking cigarettes, and drug abuse. These habits can either cause a miscarriage early on or be as severe as to induce pregnancy loss late in the pregnancy. You want to make sure that your health is up to par when you get pregnant. The glaring statistics are that a large number of pregnancies that happen are unplanned pregnancies, which means that women can often be unprepared for them. However, we can always make changes even after the first few weeks of pregnancy to try and offset any negative lifestyle habits. If you are planning on getting pregnant then begin by changing to healthy lifestyle habits sooner rather than later. Surprisingly, living in the middle of a bustling city has been shown to have a link to miscarriages due to the exposure of nitrogen dioxide. This gas will naturally be found in increased levels in the city rather than the country.

5. Other issues like blood clotting disorders can also cause miscarriages. These types of miscarriages are rare, however, they do still happen to women who particularly suffer from Factor V Leiden disorder. There is very little you can do in this instance except for working closely with your physician, and even then, it is out of your hands half the time.

6. Physical complications can come into play when uterine abnormalities such as polyps occur. Even cervical incompetence can play a role in a miscarriage. Generally, physical complication losses happen later in pregnancy but they can still happen in the first trimester.

7. Lastly, immunological disorders can lead to miscarriage. While many healthcare professionals debate the effect these disorders have on pregnancy, there is still some agreement that the autoimmune disorders that women face play a role in a miscarriage. This particularly becomes a factor in recurrent miscarriages. While it is still being researched, the simplest way to explain the connection between an autoimmune disorder and a miscarriage is that the body refuses to accept the pregnancy. For example, for women who suffer from the autoimmune disease Lupus, they could have a higher chance of miscarriage because of some of the antibodies that are present in their systems. It is recommended for women who experience recurrent miscarriages to get tested for antiphospholipid syndrome. Recurrent miscarriages are normally defined as more than three random miscarriages. While you will not be able to control the presence of these antibodies in your system, you might find a treatment that reduces the risk of miscarriage and allows you to carry to term.

How to Live With Miscarriage

Miscarriage brings with it many complicated emotions. Espccially if you were rejoicing and wanting the baby that you were expecting to carry to term. Dealing with sudden and unexpected loss can be traumatizing. The loss is not lessened by the fact that you never got to hold your baby or see it, and sometimes this can greatly impact the loss.

There is no rule book for what you can or what you should feel during this time of stress and sadness. You might find that you are slipping into behaviors that are negative like withdrawing from your loved ones. It might even be too hard for you to reach out to those who have babies because you are afraid of feeling resentment toward them. You might shed a million tears and you might shed none. There is no rhyme or rhythm, and the response you feel you need to give is the right one. Your response to your miscarriage is okay and normal.

Feelings of confusion are heightened during times of miscarriage as many women don't exactly understand everything that has happened, is happening, or what they are going to go through. It is important to understand what you are going through and your options because it can help provide some clarity to you during this dark time. It can also give you some shred of normalcy to cling to while you process your emotions.

Do you know entirely what a miscarriage is? A miscarriage happens when an embryo is pushed out from the uterus before it becomes able to survive by itself. This normally happens within the first trimester of your pregnancy. Normally, the first symptom of a miscarriage will be some back pain or abdominal cramping along with a heavy flow of blood. These symptoms can last for a few days or for a period of three weeks. It merely depends on how far along you were in your pregnancy. If at any time while pregnant you experience cramping and bleeding, go and see your physician or go to the emergency room if it is severe so that you can take the next steps toward your health.

Two things can happen when you realize you are having a miscarriage. You might be almost through with the miscarriage by the time you see a doctor, or it might not have started yet. At any time you suspect a miscarriage, you should go see your doctor. They will use an ultrasound to confirm or deny your suspicions. They might even perform a pelvic exam on you to make sure that your cervix is not dilating. There could also be some blood testing included in your appointment just to make sure that you are in good shape physically.

If you are diagnosed as having a miscarriage, the next few steps can be extremely difficult. Your uterus will need to be emptied of all that is currently occupying its space. This is because your uterus needs to make space for your menstrual cycles to resume in an attempt to prepare for fertilization again. This process depends on how many weeks into your pregnancy you were. If it was only a week or two then the bleeding you experienced could have been the complete emptying of all fetal tissue from your uterus. Unfortunately, if you are well into your first trimester, than bleeding does not complete the miscarriage because there might still be remnants of the pregnancy within your uterus. This is called an incomplete miscarriage and will have to be completed by a doctor. There is more than one way your doctor can help you facilitate the completion of your pregnancy.

1. Expectant management is where you decide that you would rather your pregnancy naturally remove itself from the body. This is where your body can take anywhere from four days to four weeks to completely expel the pregnancy remains from your body before resuming a regular menstrual cycle. Your doctor will go over all the risks of this with you and explain what you should expect before they allow you to follow through with this method.

2. Sometimes the remains of pregnancy do not want to come out on their own, or it appears as if they won't. Then your doctor can step in with medication like mifepristone which will help speed up the expulsion of the embryo. This can be taken in a pill. There is also a vaginal suppository that does the same job. You will notice that in two or three days, you start to push out the extra fetal tissue and the placenta that had formed. The length of time this can take is entirely dependent on your body and what it needs. Every woman's length of time varies. There are side effects with these medications, of course, and you might find that you go through additional bleeding, nausea, cramping, and even diarrhea while on this medication.

3. Your third option will be surgery. It is a minor surgery. Dilation and curettage (D&C) is where a doctor will scrape the placenta and the fetal remains from your uterus and ensure there are no pregnancy remains. You might still experience bleeding after this procedure, but it should clear up within a week. Sometimes (because it is surgery) there are infections that can occur as a side effect, however, this is not common.

You might be feeling overwhelmed with which choice is the right one to make. Well, sometimes your doctor can help you with this. Don't be afraid to lean on your healthcare provider during this scary time as they can guide you into the right decision for your body. The path the doctor recommends will depend on how far along the miscarriage has progressed and how severe the bleeding or cramping is. For example, if you are far into the miscarriage then your doctor might opt to have your miscarriage continue naturally. If there is cramping but no signs of bleeding then medication or surgery will be discussed.

Remember that this is not all about your physical state. You will have emotional ramifications to deal with as well. Sometimes the wait during a natural miscarriage can mentally kill you and bring your entire psychological state down. Most women won't begin to process the loss until after the full miscarriage is complete. This is why having the miscarriage process sped up can help with the recovery time.

While D&C can be invasive and brings with it rare risks for possible infection, it still helps the miscarriage be completed sooner which allows women a faster rate of mental recovery from the loss. Remember that expelling the fetal remains naturally doesn't always guarantee a hundred percent success rate. There might still be remains that have to be removed surgically. It is also far easier to pinpoint a cause for the miscarriage when a D&C is performed — though a cause is not always guaranteed.

You need to talk to your doctor about an appropriate time to dive back into regular activities. This means carrying on with your life as usual. Some routines and activities like exercise might be resumed fairly soon after a miscarriage, however, other activities like sex might come with a longer waiting period. You might even be told to abstain from using menstrual cups or condoms or inserting anything into your vagina for a period of time so that you don't get an infection. You will need a follow-up appointment with your physician when you are ready to evaluate your health after the miscarriage.

You might feel as if you do not need a follow up with your doctor after your miscarriage, but it is vital that even a few months after the miscarriage you make sure your body is working as it should. While miscarriage complications are rare, they are still something you want to keep an eye out for.

Bleeding that happens for longer than seven days might indicate that parts of the placenta remained in your uterus. It could also be a sign that an infection has developed. Look out for any discharge that smells funky and any fevers you might experience as those are also symptoms of infection. An infection of that magnitude is normally treated with antibiotics. Once in a blue moon, a woman suffers what is known as a choriocarcinoma. This is where the embryo and placenta remain in the uterus and grow together into a tumor. This is why a follow-up appointment can be critical for your health and well-being.

When the physical side of your well-being is taken care of, you have to confront the emotional side of your well-being. You will most likely experience the different stages of grief during this difficult time. No amount of wishful thinking will bring back the lost pregnancy or change your emotional state. You will need to come to terms with the loss and work towards mental and emotional healing. You might recognize some of the steps of grief, but remember that they can occur in different stages — particularly the first three.

- Denial and shock might be among the first feelings you experience. You might feel numb about the miscarriage. This is perfectly normal. These emotions exist to protect your own mind from how traumatic the loss might be to you.

- Anger and guilt can come next. You might be looking for someone to blame. It could be your partner, your doctor, but most times you end up blaming yourself. This is especially true for women who go through unplanned pregnancy miscarriages. They start to believe that they willed the baby away. Sometimes you will bring religion into it and get angry with the Deity you worship for letting you experience this pain. Sometimes anger builds up against women who are pregnant or who already have children. You might find it hard to be around them because it reminds you of your loss.

- Despair and depression come into play and you will find that you feel sad or exhausted. Negative behaviors might manifest where you stop eating and sleeping properly. You might have no desire to continue to function in your everyday life.

- Acceptance will eventually settle on you, and you will make peace with the loss. This doesn't mean that you will forget that the loss happened, but you will be able to accept that this happened in your journey of life and you will find some ways to continue to move forward.

Please do not be unconditionally hard on yourself during this phase — as difficult advice as this must be to swallow. It is normal and okay for you to experience your grief, and you have every right to your emotions. Whether you were one week or four weeks into your pregnancy, there is no rule book for how to deal with the loss of an expected baby.

Have patience with well-meaning friends. You might even hear the words, "You can try again" and these could anger you. Try to understand that your friends are not trying to hurt you, they simply do not have the words to offer you comfort.

You should find your own way to grieve. While some people find closure in a mock funeral for the baby (normally a private affair with only the mother or parents of loss taking part) others find closure by turning their attention to other activities. Remember that you cannot stay in one place forever. You have to keep trying to move forward and find closure.

It is okay and acceptable for you to sit and grieve as you need to, but you cannot stay there forever. You need to start moving on with your life. Some tips I can provide to you are:

- Don't isolate yourself. Allow your partner to be your support. They might also be grieving over the loss, and their grief might look different than yours. Talk to one another and be the foundation for each other to heal rather than turning away from each other.

- For those who hold deep religious beliefs, talking to your religious leader can help provide you some closure or guidance on how to cope with the grief.

- Find support from others going through similar issues either in person or through an online forum. There are many options for support for miscarriage.

- Reach out to a counselor or therapist who can assist you with working through the complicated emotions of miscarriage.

The surprising thing about miscarriage is that you are not alone. Over 15 percent of all pregnancies end in miscarriage. This means that there are millions of other women out there who have experienced and will experience grief and loss. Sometimes it can be a comfort to know that there are people you can reach out to that understand your feelings of sadness during this time.

You might even think that you will never feel normal again in your life. That is a fairly common feeling and belief for many people who experience a traumatic loss like a miscarriage. Nothing but time and positive work toward yourself will help you heal and move on. Sometimes positive work comes in the way of accepting that a part of your heart will always hold love for the lost pregnancy. Allow yourself to acknowledge the sadness on the anniversary dates of the baby's loss. Sometimes you can plan a special day for yourself, or even yourself and your partner, as you work through the anniversary of sadness. Find joy through this time and try to reconnect with your partner rather than push them away.

Eventually, you will find that you will start feeling better. You might never feel like your "old self" again, but you will feel different. You will feel lighter and happier, and you will realize that your ability to smile has not forsaken you. If you truly find that time is passing and you are not coping with the loss and you are battling to eat and sleep then you should reach out for professional help with your recovery journey.

One of the worst parts of experiencing a miscarriage is the idea of getting pregnant again. It is recommended that before you try to get pregnant again, you should give yourself at least three to six months to recover both physically and emotionally from the miscarriage. While you can try again fairly soon after a miscarriage (about one menstrual cycle) thanks to the body's amazing ability to heal itself, you want to give yourself time to come to terms with your loss.

However, most women do get pregnant again after a miscarriage, and it is completely possible to carry a healthy baby to full term after a miscarriage. Try and become comfortable with the idea of pregnancy again if you really do want a baby. A miscarriage is not the end to your fertility, oftentimes it is a precursor to your future fertility.

Idiopathic Infertility

Idiopathic infertility is merely unexplained infertility. This is where the reason for infertility is unknown, even after all the tests have been run to determine why a couple might be experiencing troubles getting pregnant. Testing to diagnose idiopathic infertility includes tests on the man's semen and testing out a woman's fallopian tubes and her ovulation period.

It is not unlikely that abnormalities are present with idiopathic infertility, in fact, it is a guarantee that there is an abnormality that exists. Unfortunately, the current testing methods available are unable to detect the underlying cause of infertility. Sometimes with idiopathic infertility, the woman's egg is not released in time for fertilization or the sperm might not quite reach the egg when it is ready.

There are very few answers for idiopathic infertility. Sometimes the problem resolves itself, other times other options for conception need to be discussed with the doctor.

Brief Recap

I don't want you to leave this chapter with fears in your heart, but rather with a light at the end of the tunnel that there is still hope for you to get pregnant after a miscarriage. And if you are or have experienced a miscarriage, that there is a way through all of the grief that you are experiencing. Miscarriage has a lot of information to it, but I will highlight only a few main points.

- Miscarriage happens in 15 percent of all pregnancies.

- There are three options for miscarriage: natural expulsion, medication to expel, and D&C surgery to help remove the remnants of the fetus.

- There are many medical conditions like thyroid disorders and diabetes that can impact miscarriages. Certain bad lifestyle habits can also increase the chance of a miscarriage.

- You are entitled to your grief following a miscarriage, and you might go through several different stages before you enter the stage of acceptance.

- If you have a partner, remember that you are not the only one experiencing loss during this time. Your partner could be an invaluable support to you.

- If you find yourself slipping into depression following a miscarriage, seek out professional help to aid you with your recovery.

- A miscarriage is not a marker for infertility and many women can get and do get pregnant after a miscarriage.

Chapter 9: Getting Pregnant

Okay! So, I know why you are here. You want to get pregnant. How can you maximize your fertility and get pregnant? I have already covered several different ways you could boost your fertility, but now I am going to go through the most important ways you can help yourself get pregnant. I am throwing all of my baby-making powder your way!

Maximize Fertility and Getting Pregnant

The fun fact of the day is that simply by controlling your diet and lifestyle you can increase your fertility by a whopping 69 percent!

Remember those antioxidants I was telling you about earlier? Eating foods that are rich in antioxidants is an excellent way to begin boosting your fertility because they help repair and protect your reproductive system. Their main job is to kill off the free radicals in your body that cause damage to both sperm and eggs.

This next trick might seem odd but it really does work. Eating a bigger breakfast can help you with infertility issues, particularly for women who suffer from PCOS. When you eat more calories during your breakfast meal and less calories during your evening meal, your levels of the insulin hormone are more balanced in your body.

If you don't normally exercise then you might want to start

working out those glutes! An active and healthy lifestyle often is an indicator for good fertility health. Make sure that you balance your exercise though as high levels of exercise can cause the opposite effect and leave you with infertility. Life is all about balance and you need to find yours.

There are also natural supplements you can take that are supposed to increase your fertility. For example:

Bee pollen has shown that it improves the body's immune system as well as levels of fertility. Even male fertility has shown a proven success rate with bee pollen.

Maca is found on a plant that is native to Peru. It has been shown to increase and improve the chances of reproductive success in those who take it.

There must be something fantastic about those bees because bee propolis (a mixture of beeswax and bee saliva) has shown to assist women who battle with endometriosis. In fact, it has helped women who take it two times a day increase their chances of getting pregnant by 40 percent in a time frame of 9 months.

Royal Jelly is also a product created by bees. It is filled with lipids, healthy sugars, fatty acids, amino acids, calcium, iron, and a host of vitamins that are good for us. While it is still being tested on humans, it has shown to cause improvement in the reproductive health of animals that it has been administered to.

Treatments and Tests for Getting Pregnant

If you are struggling with infertility there are other treatments you can get to raise your chances of fertility. Our medical advances have enabled us to allow women to carry to term healthy babies under many different conditions and battles with infertility.

The most common treatments for fertility are:

- In Vitro Fertilization (IVF): your eggs will be taken from your ovaries and fertilized in a lab with your chosen sperm. They develop into embryos in a lab environment and then the embryo is inserted into your uterus.

- Intrauterine Insemination (IUI): sperm is collected by your chosen donor and then inserted into your uterus during your ovulation for your best chance at getting pregnant.

These are normally used in extreme cases of infertility and they can be expensive options to explore. Make sure that you have exhausted all other routes before attempting these methods of getting pregnant and that you have discussed the possible outcomes with your doctor. Keep in mind that a healthy lifestyle still applies to IVF and IUI and can drastically increase the success rate that you have with them.

Brief Recap

Getting pregnant sometimes requires more work than letting your partner ejaculate in you and hoping his sperm fertilizes your egg. There are so many different things you can do to maximize your fertility or other options to explore when trying to get pregnant.

- IVF and IUI are medically facilitated ways of getting pregnant. A healthy lifestyle improves their success rate at implantation.

- There are a host of supplements like beeswax that you can try in order to boost your fertility. Always double-check with your healthcare provider before you start taking a new supplement though.

- Exercise and a healthy diet are your two biggest allies when it comes to boosting your fertility. Do yourself a favor and eat spinach and take a walk at least once a day!

Chapter 10: A Healthy Pregnancy

So, you did it! You got pregnant and you want to know how to maintain a healthy pregnancy! Congratulations! Or future congratulations if you are not here yet and are merely preparing for your future baby! Either way, you need to be prepared for the changes that your body is about to go through. Let's jump right into learning all about pregnancy!

How to Know When You Are Pregnant

Getting pregnant can be a very exciting time in your life. In fact, it can be joyous too. If you are on the tip of your toes waiting to see if you are pregnant, pay attention to some of these signs your body will let you know:

- If you miss a period when you normally have a regular menstrual cycle this can be the first sign of pregnancy. Keep in mind if your cycle is irregular you cannot use this sign.

- If you experience nausea. This can be with vomiting and without vomiting. Even though it is commonly called morning sickness, nausea that is associated with pregnancy can occur at any time of the day. This includes morning and night. Typically you will experience nausea a month into your pregnancy but it has been known to start sooner as well.

- Swollen breasts that are tender to the touch start early

on in pregnancy. Due to all the hormones changing in your body, your breasts will react by feeling fuller than usual and more sensitive to the touch.

- Peeing more frequently is a common symptom of pregnancy. Because you have more blood running through your body during pregnancy, your kidneys work extra hard and produce more fluid which makes you have to go to the bathroom more often.

- Fatigue is another symptom of pregnancy. It is one of the first things you will experience in the early stages of pregnancy. You will feel sleepy and might even find yourself sleeping for longer hours than you usually do.

There are other more obscure signs of pregnancy that you can go through as well. Not everyone experiences these symptoms, and they can sometimes overlap with other conditions or even your menstrual cycle. However, if you suspect that you are pregnant or are trying to get pregnant, pay attention to see if you feel:

- Moody. In the first trimester of pregnancy, your hormones are elevated and playing in your body getting it ready for a baby. These hormones will make you overly emotional and you might experience occasional mood swings.

- Light spotting can be a sign of implantation bleeding. Sometimes women mistake it for the beginning of their period. When your fertilized egg buries itself into the thickened uterine lining you can sometimes have implantation bleeding.

- Feeling bloated when you first get pregnant is common and many women mistake it as a sign of their impending menstrual cycle, however, they are really growing a baby inside them!

- Other symptoms like cramping and constipation can also happen during the first trimester. However, they overlap with many other conditions so it can be hard to pinpoint these to decipher if you are pregnant or not.

- If you feel any aversion to specific foods this can indicate that you might be pregnant. When pregnant, you become hypersensitive to certain scents and your taste buds might change on you. Suddenly a food you loved you hate and vice versa!

So, are you really pregnant? While these symptoms are great ways to test if you might be in the early stages of pregnancy and they can be fun to look out for when you are trying to conceive, the best way to test for pregnancy is to use an at-home kit.

When you get a positive reading on an at-home pregnancy test then you should make an appointment with your healthcare provider so that they can confirm your results! It is helpful to know as soon as possible so that you can start the appropriate regimen of prenatal care for your baby!

What Your Body Will Go Through When Pregnant

As you go through pregnancy, you can't expect your body to remain the same. There will be a lot of changes that your body will undergo to prepare for the growing baby.

You might be surprised at the changes such as bleeding gums. Many women have a problem with bleeding gums that leave them open to infections in the mouth while expecting. It's important you keep up with your oral health to lessen the impact of bleeding gums.

During pregnancy, you might find that your hair is looking better than ever. Your hormones during pregnancy will stimulate hair growth — not simply on your head but everywhere! Your nails might also get more brittle as your pregnancy progresses.

Don't be shocked if you find stretch marks appearing on your body. These are often a common and unwelcome bodily change your skin goes through for pregnancy. This is because your skin has to stretch to accommodate your growing body.

Have you looked at your nipples lately? The area around a woman's nipple called the areola will often darken, and at times expand, during pregnancy.

The other bodily change you might notice is that you sweat a lot more during pregnancy because your body temperature is higher than before.

Diet and Exercise While Pregnant

Many people become concerned when they get pregnant that exercise is not a good option for them. However, exercise during pregnancy is safe and actually recommended! Especially if you were physically active before you got pregnant. You should always discuss your exercise with your doctor, but as long as it is safe and you have no other pressing health issues, you should be able to exercise right through your pregnancy.

You don't want weight loss to be your main goal with exercise, but merely maintaining a healthy lifestyle. Exercise is not only used for weight loss but to keep your body functioning as it should and also for that release of endorphins that you get. In fact, there are all sorts of exercises catered to pregnant women like prenatal yoga!

When you exercise appropriately during pregnancy you can find benefits such as:

- Increased energy
- Prevention of gestational diabetes
- A reduction in back pain and bloating
- An improved mood
- Better sleep at night
- Improved muscles and tone of your body. It also helps prepare your body for the activity during labor.

When you are pregnant, partaking in a healthy lifestyle is critical. You can take all the prenatal vitamins and supplements that you want, however, these are only supposed to complement a healthy diet. You can negatively impact your health and your baby's growth if you do not eat a well-balanced diet from the main food groups.

While you are pregnant, you should eat at least four servings of vegetables and two servings of fruit. These foods provide you a ton of nutritional support in the form of vitamins and folic acid as well as antioxidants.

Eating bread and healthy grains like quinoa will help increase your fiber and also support your nutrition needs during your pregnancy. Eating between 6 to 10 ounces of grains every day is vital to your growing pregnancy needs.

You must maintain a good amount of calcium intake, about 1000mg every day. Full-fat milk and creams and cheeses are a good place to find the calcium that is needed to support your growing baby and yourself. Remember that whatever your baby needs to grow, it will take it from you, and you then have to replenish your own stock of nutrients or you can suffer from bad health.

Brief Recap

It is no secret that healthy eating and exercise are important to a woman during pregnancy, but did any of those bodily changes catch you unaware?

- Stretch marks are common occurrences across your skin as your body enlarges to make room for the baby growing within you.

- Continuing to exercise while pregnant is vital if you exercised before you were pregnant. Maintaining good health can see you through a happy and healthy pregnancy.

- Your hair growth will increase while you are pregnant which will give you a lot of great hair days, but you might find unexpected hair growth in unwanted places.

Conclusion

Congratulations, we covered a lot in this book . Confronting issues related to fertility and pregnancy can be a scary topic for most women to broach, and I am proud of you for completing this. I hope that the information that you have learned from this guide can be carried with you as you carry on with your journey.

Your journey will vary from others that read this book, and everyone has their own reason as to why they picked it up. Some women simply want to know more about their bodies and the way that they work, while other women might be getting ready to enter the stage of trying for a baby.

If you are a woman who has suffered through miscarriage and loss and has turned to this book as a comfort and a "where do I go from here?" guide then I offer you up nothing but my sincerest and warmest wishes. I know you are going through some dark times, but pay attention to those chapters that offer hopeful words about life before and after miscarriage. We are all a part of the same journey in this world, we simply lead our journeys in different ways.

At the end of the day, you need to find comfort within your own body and locate an ability to interact with yourself intimately. This is vital because as you track your body and its changes, you will need to be able to feel comfortable with touching parts of yourself like your cervix or your vaginal lips. There are also monthly breast exams that you should conduct yourself to ensure that your health is in optimal shape.

Charting can give a woman a huge sense of body autonomy. You will know when something is wrong and whether it is the cause of a decision you made earlier in the week or a marker that you need to go to your doctor and get examined. Your body is with you every single day waiting and hoping for you to unlock your true understanding of it.

You have now read all the guided chapters that I have to offer you on your body and your fertility. You should now know from chapters one to three exactly how to chart and what signs you need to keep track of to chart your fertile and infertile periods. How crazy is it that you only have a 12-24 hour window of getting pregnant every month? Your newfound abilities at charting will help you find this window of fertility. If you are using methods of natural family planning then you know when you need to use condoms and/or the pull out method (although the pull out method is not recommended as it only has a 70 percent success rate). If you are hoping to conceive then charting will help you make the most of your window of fertility. I find that one of the greatest benefits from charting is that you are able to keep track of your fertility and not take the fun out of the bedroom for you or your partner.

As you delved deeper into this guide, I know you have been armed with knowledge about your diet and the effect that it has on your body. Regardless of your plans for conception, it is important to know what foods might negatively affect your body and what foods will nourish your body. When it comes to fertility, being aware of your food is vital, and you should make the necessary changes as soon as possible if you are trying to conceive.

There are so many health choices we make that affect the way our bodies and hormones react, oftentimes without us being aware that we are negatively affecting ourselves. The last thing I would want for you is the difference between fertility and infertility to be a lack of knowledge.

You can do this. You can take control of your life and your fertility. The statistics and information imparted in this guide prove that you can! I want you to walk away from this guide with a sense of accomplishment and empowerment. Yes, some of the information might have been scary to confront. Some of it might have been heartbreaking. However, you did it. You faced it. You learned it, and now all that is left to do is for you to apply it.

You are the master of your own world and life. For those of you women reading this who have the ultimate goal of getting pregnant, chapters nine and ten should have imparted to you the most vital information you can take with as you enter this incredible journey.

Infertility can be difficult to deal with. So many months, and cycle after cycle you can begin to feel useless and out of control. I want you to change that feeling for yourself. We throw thousands of dollars at healthcare professionals to inspect our bodies and tell us what is wrong with us, what's wrong with buying a 99 cent calendar and pen to track our own body's changes? It will cost you virtually nothing to track your body's menstrual cycle and physical changes every month.

By learning to take control of your body and your life, you lose nothing and you gain everything. What's the saying... "What do you have to lose?" I can honestly promise you that the only thing you will lose when you take a vested interest in your body and reproductive system is the unhealthy habits that you have formed over a lifetime of being fed misinformation.

You see, the time is not later today, or tomorrow, or next week. No. The time for you to initiate change is right this second. Right now. As you turn the last page of this guide and you sit there with any notes or thoughts that are musing in your mind, you should spring into action the change that you wish to see in your life.

I have fulfilled my promise to you. I told you I would give you the power to understand your body and to predict changes in your body before your doctors can. Now, the only person standing in your way is you. You are armed with knowledge. You are armed with the necessary tools. You have everything you need to enact change.

My parting words to you as you digest the wealth of information within these chapters are that I hope you find success in charting your cycle and managing your fertility. If you are struggling with infertility now, I hope this guide has given you solace and options for where to turn to next. Happy charting ladies!

Reference List

Berry, J. (2017). Anovulation: Symptoms, causes, and treatment. Retrieved 12 November 2019, from https://www.medicalnewstoday.com/articles/318552.php

Brazier, Y. (2017). Irregular periods: Symptoms, causes, home remedies, and treatment. Retrieved 12 November 2019, from https://www.medicalnewstoday.com/articles/178635.php

Brusie, C. (2019). https://www.parents.com. Retrieved 12 November 2019, from https://www.parents.com/pregnancy/complications/miscarriage/top-7-causes-of-miscarriage/

Eur Neuropsychopharmacol. 2014 Nov;24(11):1855-9. doi: 10.1016/j.euroneuro.2014.08.015. Epub 2014 Sep 1.

Int J Environ Res Public Health. 2019 Jul 30;16(15). pii: E2723. doi: 10.3390/ijerph16152723.

Johnson, M. (2010). Can't Get Pregnant? How Stress May Be Causing Your Infertility. Retrieved 12 November 2019, from https://health.usnews.com/health-news/family-health/womens-health/articles/2010/08/27/cant-get-pregnant-how-stress-may-be-causing-your-infertility

Obos Anatomy. (2014). Charting Your Menstrual Cycle - Our Bodies Ourselves. Retrieved 12 November 2019, from https://www.ourbodiesourselves.org/book-excerpts/health-article/charting-your-menstrual-cycle/

Vigil, P., Blackwell, L. F., & Cortés, M. E. (2012). The Importance of Fertility Awareness in the Assessment of a Woman's Health a Review. The Linacre quarterly, 79(4), 426–450. doi:10.1179/002436312804827109

Weiss, S. (2019). 9 Foods to Avoid If You're Trying to Get Pregnant. Retrieved 12 November 2019, from https://www.glamour.com/story/foods-to-avoid-if-youre-trying-to-get-pregnant

www.ingramcontent.com/pod-product-compliance
Lightning Source LLC
Chambersburg PA
CBHW030712220526
45463CB00005B/2018